ALL THE SIGNS OF BRAIN DAMAGE

THE RELATIONSHIP CHRONICLES

The "Getting to Know" Process

TONEE MORTON

First published by Dog Ear Publishing
4010 W. 86th Street, Ste H
Indianapolis, IN 46268
www.dogearpublishing.net

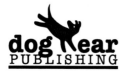

ISBN: 978-1-4575-1591-0

This book is printed on acid-free paper.

Printed in the United States of America

Being alone only prepares you for one thing... and that is *being alone.*

ACKNOWLEDGEMENTS

To my Mom:

I know that you are looking down on me wondering what the heck I was thinking writing this book without you being here to protect me. Well mom, you are here protecting me. And every day that I wake up, I feel your presence in my life because you have taught me so much. And loving you and appreciating you for everything that you have meant to me is not something that I take lightly. I am happy that you are with GOD. I just wish he would allow you to come back and talk to me every once in a while.

To My Children:

I know that I have not always been there in person, but I never stopped loving and thinking about you. I have always prayed and asked GOD to keep you protected while I go and make a life for you. And now that it's complete, daddy is coming for you—to be there helping you with your relationships with the opposite sex and trying to be a role model in your development as you search for the "love" that I have always had for you guys. I just hope that you could be as proud of me as I am of you.

To All my family:

I know that it has been a hard road since the elders of our dominion have passed and we all have gone our separate ways to raise our immediate families. I just want to thank all of you who have thought or wondered about me as I have thought and wondered about you. There isn't a day that goes by that I don't think about all the good times that I had as a child with you and all the good times that we are going to have being laborers of children. Until then, just know that I have never forgotten about any of you. I love you!

To the World:

Thank you for showing me that through all the trials and tribulations, bad news and destruction, poverty and suffering—that people still carry a sense of love and responsibility to more than themselves. Thank you for showing me that the heart still beats for the incline of man rather than the decline. Thank you for allowing me to see first hand the things we are capable of doing when we see our differences as strengths and not weaknesses. What a pleasure it has been to be a part of history!

Table of Contents

Prologue

As far back as I can remember, my mom always said that men got "brain damage" and women got "dain bramage." And it could not be more evident than it is today. From the moment I started dating to the time that I realized I was too old to be dating, I knew that I was not approaching my interactions with women in the same manner that my stepfather did with my mother and my grandfather did with my grandmother. Something was missing, and I wanted to find out what it was. So instead of embarking on a relationship expedition that may have been able to give me some of the answers I was looking for—or depend upon best sellers written by people who have been in less relationships than a gay guy in a straight bar—I decided that it was time for me to try and figure it out for myself, as well as those of *you* who have been searching for answers.

One of the things that always rang true about any and every situation I encountered is that I had lost my perspective of what it took to be in a relationship right from the start because I didn't acknowledge the "getting to know" process for what it was. I realized that I made this process "null and void" in my own pursuit of relationships and the way that I was suppose to be in those relationships. The ignorance that I displayed in the getting to know process put me at a disadvantage—because I didn't realize that this aspect would "make" or "break" the relationship. Ironically, by the time I came to my senses about what I was looking for in a woman, I was going back and forth in my mind to try and figure out how my approach to the getting to know process pertained to my previous relationships. It was a staggering admission to acknowledge that my way of doing things, or not doing things, had contributed to all of my failed attempts at true love.

I created part of the chaos and mayhem that became a huge part of my life because I had been brainwashed by the men around me who had given me the indication that the getting to know process was not that important. I had even been brainwashed into thinking that the getting to know process was about me. But it wasn't! It was about the women that I had dealt with to tell me what and how they needed things done in order for us to be happy in the routine part of our relationship.

But when you have all the signs of brain damage, as a man or a woman, you go into the **"getting to know "** process creating an issue that doesn't exist because your insecurities won't allow you to enjoy what is natural and pleasing about the person you're trying to be with. When you have all the signs of brain damage, you go out and sabotage your chance with Mr. Right or Ms. Right because you sat and watched a show about relationships that had nothing to do with you or where you wanted to be with your future mate. Yes! I was the birth child of brain damage and some of you are as well. I had allowed the opinions and examples created by other people for themselves to make its way into my life. Never once did I question the validity of my own desires to be who I wanted to be for the person who deserved it.

I made a mess of all of my attempts at love, and so have you, my friend! So many of you out there in the world today are making a big mistake trying to be in a relationship where you have made a mockery of the **getting to know** process. You have treated this process as a mute point as to what you think is important—and that would ultimately be developing a loving relationship with a wonderful partner! That's where you think it will all turn around for you, but it won't as long as you continue to ignore the fact that *"failing to prepare a man or a woman to be in your life is preparing them to fail in the relationship"*.

So! In an effort to keep others from making the same mistakes that I did along the way, I made the decision that it was time for me to challenge the real status quo and find out where this brain-damaged way of thinking began: **OURSELVES!** Now, I'm not saying that this process is going to be a pleasant experience by any means! I'm not saying that what I have written is going to agree with your spirit. I'm not even promising that this book is going to make it's way into Oprah Winfrey's book club! But what I am saying is this—if you allow yourself to be honest with these words, then they will be honest with you. Otherwise, you have just wasted your money on this book and I am not giving it back. (SMILE) The money that is…the advice is yours to keep for free!

CHAPTER 1

"The Getting to Know Process"

So many times in the getting to know process—men and women tend to depend on everyone and everything to give them a sense of how they should approach one another in this process. Everything from the magazine racks to your favorite morning show, all the way to your closest friends and your favorite relationship book, you have been given the blueprint as to how you should be getting to know each other. The trouble with that is most men and women only think about the reward and never the consequence of how the getting to know process is presented and/or played out. Most of the time as men and women you think that your main goal is to get this person to like you, when your primary goal should be getting this person to respect the fact that you are bringing your own individuality to the table.

When I started doing my research to uncover the ways in which human beings went about getting to know each other, one of the things that I found myself realizing was even though society has created more ways and methods that are making the "meet and greet process" easier, it did not necessarily give us a more definitive way of making the getting to know process more *effective*. In fact, when I think about all of the devices that have been created to help men and women communicate (i.e., cell phones, computers, emailing and text messaging), I feel that our interaction with one another has declined, not improved. As a society, we are no closer to making the getting to know process run more smoothly than when Thomas Edison was alive, because no matter how much technology society creates to make the introduction process to the opposite sex easier, the human element still applies when trying to make that connection. So now the question becomes more about the way in which we go about communicating more than the communication itself.

Like most people I have started doing most of my interacting with the opposite sex over the internet and the other devices that have been created in the past decade which only confirms that I, too, have bought into this way of communicating as well). And I have to admit that it has made my social life more like a who's who than a for sure, what is, because it had become more about sitting in front of my computer talking to people instead of actually going out and meeting with them. And dealing with the opposite sex who feels the same way as I do, doesn't seem like it's going to be a "match made in heaven" more than a "heaven knows what's going to happen." Yes! I, like most of the people on the internet, have taken the getting to know process and made it null and void to the humanistic way of doing things. And for a man who knows that women have the upper hand in the getting to know process, this doesn't make me feel much for going out of my way for a woman—especially when a woman is telling me and the rest of the world that…

"She's happy being on her own"

It's unfortunate that any woman would say that she is happy being on her own; and yet, I hear it more often than I care to admit. So I am here to say that every day that you're alone is a day that God is unsatisfied because he doesn't get to play a part in the development of your relationships. Everyday that you're alone is a day less that you will have the support from a mate who cares about your well-being. Everyday that you are alone—you die to the possibility of love ever finding you or you finding love. Everyday that you are alone is a day that you don't get to influence someone else's mind and heart to know that you will always be there for them; or that the sole reason for your existence was meant for them to benefit so that God could be pleased with your position and his.

You sabotage your own right to have what God has always presented as a priority for you because you just don't think that he was ever listening. But he was! You wanted answers for the reasons why you have never found someone or they have never found you. But it is not God's *voice* that is making up excuses about love ever finding you. It was yours! It was never God's lack of desire to want love for you more than it was your lack of desire to want love for yourself. You've had it all wrong. For the longest time you have used your tone and temperament to stir up the most gentle of crowds when you could have been using it to tame the man you claim to have been looking for all your life. You have even made excuses for your calling as a "potential mate" because you feel that although the rewards could be great, the hurt could be greater, especially if it doesn't work out. Therefore, you turn to the one thing that you think doesn't make you look helpless, which is the notion that you can use being an independent woman as your scapegoat.

But you're not happy being on your own. You're just happy that you can accept the failure in it. You even have your friends join in convincing you that you're better off without love because they know nothing about it. And even though you have a greater chance at finding love than anybody else, you settle on other people's opinions about love and take them on as your own. In the truest sense of the word, "misery loves company". Not only are you listening to your friends as you both accept this ignorance in your lives, but more than likely, they were actually hoping that you would show *them* what love was all about. So it should be disheartening that you haven't taken your place amongst the great relationships that you know about. It should be disheartening that you don't call on your heart more than your mind to make that decision for you! It should be even more disheartening that you continue to keep a mindset that the people around you will suffer from!

So you tell me how frustrating it must be to know that you have gone your entire life without ever knowing this love because you continue to be afraid of it? When are you going to say enough is enough to complacency? When are you going to throw yourself at the mercy of its courtship? There are people watching you making excuses about this love ever existing because you won't allow yourself to be vulnerable to it. This is why no man is taking the initiative to know you and connect to you because he sees the FEAR! He hears it when you speak! He can feel it when you're in his presence. That is why this other communication of emailing and text messaging has taken over because it allows you along with the rest of society to hide behind your devices and not have people seeing the negativities of your experiences first hand. But how else would there ever be a connection between men and women if neither one of us took some kind of initiative?

Therefore, I decided that it was time for me to take on this initiative of going back to the way things used to be when men and women actually got to know each other through interaction rather than emails and text messages. And so! I moved away from my computer screen in hopes of embarking upon this expedition called socializing because there was really no other way to get the answers I was looking for. However, before I could get an answer I had to know what question and/or questions needed to be answered. With that being said and with the help of a few friends, I decided to tackle one of the biggest mysteries of all:

"How do you actually get to know someone?"

Before I start feeding you and the rest of the world with the concepts I learned while doing my research for this book, I can honestly say that I wasn't one of those men who was willing to do whatever it took to get to know a woman. I mean *really* get to know her! As a matter of fact, when I look back on it now as a 41-year-old male, I realize that this concept was almost non-existent to me. I, like most men had written the getting to know process off as a mute point to what I thought was important, which is the relationship part. It wasn't until I started writing this book that I understood the importance of truly getting to know a woman, and vice versa! I just thought that I could cliff note my way through this process and expect to make up for it with my effort and attentiveness in the relationship. I also realized that most women expected for me and/or every other man to automatically know how to meet their needs in a relationship when we haven't been told what is expected of us in the getting to know process. Never once did I, or most of you for that matter, acknowledge that what was being done in the getting to know process would later become the blueprint for the relationship itself!

Like most men, I was failing at this process—thinking that I could just pick up good habits in the relationship to replace the bad habits I displayed in the getting to know process. And I am not alone! There are even a lot of women that are allowing men to come with bad habits at the start thinking that it's going to get better in the relationship. Even when women have told me straight out that **"you need to get to know me first,"** did I merely take that as her way of saying that I needed to get her comfortable enough to have sex with me. Not realizing that this was supposed to be the time for me to learn how to meet her needs correctly, so that if we did decide to take things further into a relationship—I could make the transition with no problem.

I also realized that a lot of women saying this didn't even realize that this was the most vital part of telling a man how he needs to learn how to meet their needs. Even when I have told women that they have the right to expect men to help make the transition from the getting to know process to a relationship easier, do they still hesitate in doing so. But I've got to tell you that not everything is lost in translation. You just have to know….

What person are you bringing to the table?

What person are you bringing to the table when you meet someone that you want to take things further with? This is the time to be honest with yourself and to know that the person you are bringing to the table is going to be the one that makes or breaks you and the so-called relationship you claim to be ready for. Because whether you like it or not, this is the person you are going to be stuck with being in the long run—so make it good. I would say that this is one of the most important concepts from the start because men and women are trying to figure out how their personalities are going to connect. I would compare it to the relationship between a wireless router and a computer: a) the woman being the wireless router b) the man being the computer. If you as the wireless router are giving off a bad signal, then how can a man (as the computer) connect to you? He can try as many ways possible to try and connect, but if you don't know what person you are at the time then how can he know what person he needs to be in order for the two of you to connect to each other?

So you truly have to know what person you are bringing to the table. Are you bringing a person with no issues to the table? Or do you have some questions about some things that bother you about you? Are you bringing a person who has been hurt by a woman or a man? Or are you a person who has moved beyond all that you have been through and is ready to move on? Are you bringing a person who is truly ready for something serious? Or are you a person who feels that you will show that side of yourself when someone shows you that they are just as serious? Are you bringing a person who has been single for a long time to the table and really don't know the first thing about getting yourself back into the dating scene? Or are you a person who is reinventing themselves for someone to appreciate the new you? Are you bringing a person with some flaws that you feel you need to work on? Or are you waiting on the person that you think will overlook all of those flaws and not treat them as such a big deal?

Are you bringing a person with a troubled past that you're afraid to discuss? Or are you the kind of person who is not afraid of the backlash that is going to come from the bad decisions you've made in your life? Are you bringing a person that needs a man or a woman in your life to blame? Or are you the kind of person who will take responsibility for your part in the relationship? Are you bringing a person that claims to be set in their ways? Or are you accepting the fact that being so-called set in those ways is making you look like a person who is selfish and not willing to compromise? Are you bringing a person that is still dealing with childhood issues? Or are you dealing with those issues so that you don't burden a total stranger with issues they had nothing to do with? Are you bringing a person who feels the world owes them something? Or are you accepting the fact that you have not earned your right to expect anything and therefore don't deserve it? Are you bringing a person who is okay being alone? Or are you accepting this as being in denial of your own desire to mate because you have failed at it and the disappointment is too great to continue putting yourself out there? Are you bringing a so-called independent person to the table? Or are you starting to realize that being that way is stopping you from allowing someone to love you and make things easier for you? Or are you bringing to the table a person that deep down inside doesn't believe that **"LOVE"** will ever find them?

These were some of the questions that I asked myself once upon a time, and some of you are still asking these questions today. Who are you when you are presenting yourself to a man or a woman? Even when I wasn't asking myself this question when I would meet a woman—I always knew it in the back of my mind what person I was bringing to the table. And I'm sure you know as well. At times I didn't want to admit that I was bringing a tainted soul to the table but my conscience wouldn't allow me not to acknowledge it for being there. So many times I thought that I could work my way through these issues by not acknowledging them. But that became the sole reason why things went wrong in the "getting know process" and never would make its way to the so-called relationship part of this equation. As I look back on those situations in my own life one of the things that became very evident to me is that...

"My conscience did have a way of showing my denial its true colors through all my failed attempts at love."

My conscience had a way of showing me that by not acknowledging the fact that I had brought a tainted soul to the table, I was never going to be in anything successful. That I was always going to suffer.

And you are always going to suffer as well. There are so many of you bringing a person to the table who is not ready for something real and authentic. And yet you push these elements on those who come with the realness of their heart hoping and wishing that they would make an exception on behalf of a heart that is tainted. But it is a tactic that more than likely is going to backfire on you every time because….

"Your belief system will have you at odds with your desires."

There are so many of you who are bringing a person to the table under false pretences expecting other people to over look the fact that you have tainted their abilities to present the real them. You have worked your way up the ladder to loneliness making excuses along the way to justify being the person that you are. Your reality has become more about your experiences than your desires, as you unintentionally sabotage the possibility of anyone ever appreciating being with you. Somewhere in your mindset, you believe that people care about your experiences more than your desires because you think this gives you the best chance to make your case on why you haven't found someone or are currently alone. You think that bringing this tainted person to the table will let you off the hook if something goes wrong. That's why you're not presenting the best version of yourself from the start because this part of you is not the strongest part of you! And you know that you won't be able to handle the results if the real you is not accepted by the opposite sex.

"The best version of you has taken a backseat to the person you have created to protect the other one."

And that's sad because God knows what he has in you and what you are worthy of. But you can't get beyond society's interpretations to see that you deserve something good in your life. You can't see that you have allowed other people to speak for your desires too long. So now it becomes more about the person you're not, as opposed, to the person you really are that is stopping you from benefiting the way you should be. I mean…. How can anyone satisfy you when you haven't brought your authentic self to the table? How can anyone satisfy you when you have brought a counterfeit image of who you are trying to benefit from the *real* them? The world would have you think that they will run when they see the real you, and that may well be true about most. But you're not looking for most. You're only looking for the **"ONE"** who has the capacity to accept the real you. And they will! Men will accept the real you if you just believe that you are worthy of being accepted. And women will follow suit….

Oftentimes, I have seen some of the best men and women bringing the altered image of themselves to the table because they were afraid to put the real them at risk. Not realizing they were not only putting themselves in danger but anyone wanting to get to know them as well. So many of you are putting yourselves at a disadvantage, because the real you is not being seen and appreciated by the person you desire. And now the real you is left out in the cold because the altered version that you've created was supposed to be a "beyond a reasonable doubt" representation of the real you. A slam dunk! But it isn't! You have used the backup plan as the major plan and failed. And when that happens, you can't tell the person that wasn't sold on the fake you—that now you're bringing the real one to the table. Some of you have even convinced yourselves that you like the person that you have created more than the real you because you think that this gives you the best chance right now, instead of the person that is going to last the test of time.

So what is it that you are telling yourself that is stopping you from bringing the real you to the table when looking for love? Who are you listening to? And why do you allow the real you to conjure up a false sense of who you are because you're afraid that a potential partner would not appreciate your honesty? Bringing the altered version of yourself to the table instead of the real you has become the theme song to your life—that somehow you're not good enough for someone. But in reality, you are more than good enough and have always been more than good enough. Society has sold you a bad dream that you have not woken from. You have even gone as far as to use your childhood as a scapegoat to this reality because you think that you have created in yourself an excuse prone alibi when it was never an issue before. Most would have you thinking that it made you who you are today, instead of telling you that you have always had the ability to change it. Yes! You have become the product of your own sabotage. But you don't have to be that way.

"You don't have to settle for the lesser you to satisfy the least in someone else"

You have devoted your whole life to being someone else while everyone around you has benefited from being who they really are. They know if you brought the real you to the table, they wouldn't have a chance being in your presence because they know that you're light would shine brighter. That's why they keep you believing in interpretations and opinions that have nothing to do with you. But you haven't been able to see the real you in a long time because you put that person in the closet behind the mirror you look at everyday. That's why you can't reflect the real you back to you. But no one has deserved the recognition more than you. No one has deserved someone acknowledging the real you more than you. So why the constant struggle with yourself? Why the constant questions about who you're really suppose to be when you know who you are? You know more good things about yourself than bad. So what person are you bringing to the table when you're getting to know someone? Once you identify the person you are bringing the table, most would think that this process of getting to know someone would get easier. However, nothing could be further from the truth. Especially for those women of today who are presenting themselves to men with this concept of.....

"I'm an independent woman"

Throughout the years, I have become quite familiar with the concepts that women throw at men. And I do find it fascinating that many of you have ever gotten your needs met at all. This concept has been the one that I have dissected the most since I have begun writing this book. I have had women use this phrase on their profiles on the internet. I have read this phrase used by authors in their relationship books. I have even heard this concept used by women in movies and songs. And with that, I find myself asking… has anyone ever told these women to stop telling men that they're independent and don't need a man? That they are not only taken away man's responsibility to them, but his greatest satisfaction and reward by saying this stuff? Evidently the answer is no. And you wonder why every man you meet is taking your approach for granted.

I hear women saying that they've never used the "independent" line or their friends have never used it. But what most women don't realize is there are a lot of women who are speaking for you in this instance. I mean… how could you stand by and let the women who are using this phrase give men a false sense of responsibility that has tainted the dating scene and the getting to know process? You don't realize that the more a man hears a woman saying that she's independent and doesn't need a man to do anything for her, the more he thinks that every woman he encounters feels the same way.

I mean... Beyonce practically made this phrase a household name in her song "Independent Woman." In addition, the artist Neyo followed this concept with his own song, "Ms. Independent." Now, for those of you who think that **Neyo** was agreeing with your independence, I can honestly say to you as a man—that was not the way we took it. As a matter of fact, if you stop and really listen to the lyrics, the way we took it as men is…

"You go girl! Spend your money paying your own bills, getting your hair and nails done and burning up your own account instead of mine. And when you're done using up your resources let me know so I can come over and get my needs met even though I didn't do anything to deserve it."

Yes! Neyo, much like every other man in your life, has just made a mockery of your independence without you even knowing it. And all this time you and every woman in America thought that men were being sensitive to you and every other woman's approach! In the past, I have explained to women that telling a man that you don't need him to do anything for you only presents him with the opportunity to get out of any responsibility he was looking forward to having. However, this statement doesn't seem to get through because some women are set in their ways. In fact, most women can't even see beyond their own ignorance because their defense for saying this is…

"That's not actually what I meant when I said that I didn't need a man. What I meant was…I just don't need a man to pay my bills."

This statement only makes the situation with a man worse—which is why I'm baffled that so many women continue to use the independent phrase. The other reason women have told me that they often use this phrase is because it is a defense mechanism against being hurt by men. But as women, what you must understand is that you are the ones who are creating this monster that you are considering as a "potential mate" before he even has the opportunity to establish a relationship with you. As men, they know the guy you were dealing with before them did not live up to the billing. That doesn't mean that you have to keep the next guy from living up to the billing because the guy you just got rid of couldn't do it or decided against it. Especially when he is every bit as ready to meet your needs than the knucklehead you keep talking about.

Now this independent thing would totally make sense if you were trying to be in a relationship with yourself. And I, and the other responsible men would not have a problem with it. But you don't realize how this approach has you and your female counterparts doing just that—having you in a relationship with you, yourself and no one! You don't realize how this thinking stops you from getting your needs met because you think that having this approach impresses a man. But it does no such thing. And contrary to belief, it really stops a man from wanting to take his time to invest in you. So let me be the first to tell you that…

"a man who does not invest in you is not sticking around anyway."

Now I have had women tell me that the other reason why they say that they're an "independent woman" to men is so that men don't think that they are after their money and they don't want to be considered a "gold digger." So you let him off the hook just to prove a point that will ultimately leave you frustrated and confused? You have allowed a man who doesn't know his place in your life to decide on his own how he is going to be in your life? That's not even logical or smart. Even if you try and explain to a man after the fact what you actually meant by saying this, it doesn't matter because he already has it in his head that he can play on your independence. And to a man who is looking for an excuse to be irresponsible, this is music to his ears.

And if you women think that a man is going to fight you for the position of making things easier for you that was given to him from the start, you are sadly mistaken. He will do no such thing because he knows that not fighting you for his position to make things easier for you, doesn't stop him from benefiting anyway. You being an independent woman is not going to stop him from sleeping with you, running up your light and water bill when he comes over, playing video games on the tv you bought and doing all the other things he shouldn't be given permission to do because….

"You have become so obsessed with proving your "INDEPENDENCE", that you bypass his true "MOTIVES" about your independence".

I mean…. why would I, or any other man for that matter, use our energy to try and change your perception of something that allows us to benefit even more? That's like cutting our noses off to spite our face. Why wouldn't we use your independence to our advantage? Right! But I am not here to discourage you. I am here to encourage those of you who want to see men doing better by you, to start seeing that you need to be better with your approach with them. I mean… did you know that when most men meet you for the first time, they are willing to be taught by you as to how you wanted your particular needs met?

"That their intention from the start was not to take you for granted before you presented them with the blueprint to do so."

He was in an agreeable state of mind when he first met you. And this is the thing you present him with? The "independent woman" approach? You couldn't have given him a worse thing to agree with you on. And here comes the real kick in the head! Man, even though he should be offended by this approach, he couldn't be happier because while you were trying to validate your lack of neediness, he was trying to figure out how he was going to get *his* needs met without you eventually coming to your senses. And with that, he goes on about the "relationship" doing as little as possible to be in your world. Doing just enough for you not to realize that he is not doing much at all. You don't recognize it at first because you're too busy being patted on the back by your girlfriends who think that he's some great guy just because he's taken you out on a couple of dates. But in reality, that pales in comparison as to what he's going to get out of you in the long run. However, you did get your wish. You have become the woman that all of your friends want to be like—a DIVA—which quite simply stands for:

D. I. V. A. (Dumb In Various Areas)

After four or five months of dating, you realize that the man who used to wine and dine you is now having you pay for dinner and the movie. The man that you once adored for giving you that independence is now being shown the door for reasons and excuses he didn't create. He only gave you what you originally asked for: your *independence.* This man, who took your own words of being an "independent woman" and used them against you is now being ridiculed by you and your girlfriends. And you take great delight in bringing up what you think is the obvious: that he was just an irresponsible man. But never once did you or your friends take a true inventory of how the "independent woman" approach ruined your relationship because you were too busy male bashing him into the ground instead of asking yourself, "What role did I play in this equation" so that I don't keep setting myself up to fail with men.

But how can you learn how to be successful with men when no one has ever told you to stop telling men you're an independent

15

woman? How can you learn when no one has ever told you that man will use your words against you just as much or if not more than you use his words against him? How can you learn when you claim to have been raised to do these things on your own and only incorporate a man when you want him to compliment your independence? How can you learn when the world has given you a false sense of yourself and what really makes you a woman. And I know what your arguments are going to be, or better yet, what they have been. And that is the sole definition of *want* and *need*. I hear women all the time justifying their independence by their interpretation of what want and need is, and how it pertains to their situation. And I have to say that….

"As a man I can totally understand how it would be difficult for me to come along and tell you that men don't really agree with your independence and have you accept the truth about it."

I can totally understand how it would feel if something that I used to empower myself as a man was now being brought to my attention as the sole reason why I wasn't getting my needs met by a woman. I thought most women knew that a *real* man never takes for granted a real woman's desires when they are presented in a way that pleases a man. And no! I'm not referring to a woman who is being emotional without a sense of control. That's not being vulnerable…that's being psycho! As women, you should know that a man is going on the definition of the word "independent" while you are going on the interpretation of the word "independent". As women, you should know that man takes your words literally even though you're saying them in a non-literal way. You should also know that men don't know how to separate one thing from the other because we have what I call a "present moment state of mind." So if you tell a man you don't need him for one thing, to him it means you don't need him for anything. If you tell them that you don't need them to pay your bills, men take it as you don't need them for cutting grass, buying pedicures and mani-cures, etc.

Yes! Men have taken this simple concept and used it to their advantage! And all the while women have been complaining about men's irresponsibility without realizing that they themselves were the catalyst for it. Contemplate this for a moment! Why would any man go out of his way to tell you that you are setting yourself up to be mad and disappointed in the long run because you couldn't see the dam-age you were creating? Why would a man use his energy trying to convince you that the "independent" concept will never work for you—when as a man it *is* working for him? Why would a man take away his benefit to satisfy a position you won't be appreciative of? Most of you tell men that you are ready for something serious. And yet you present men with this independent approach that make them feel like there is no possible way that they will get serious with you because their chances of being successful are little to none.

Therefore, I leave you with this—it is not a man's responsi-bility to make sure that he does not take your words and actions out of context, even though he may give you the respect in not doing so. That's your job. It's not a man's job to convince you that he should see you as more than a one night stand. That is your job as well. It is also your job to convince a man that he should be taking advantage of all your qualities. And that once you have made all of this available to him, that there is still more where that came from. Yes, the courting process does and *should* give a woman the indication that a man doesn't see her as a one night stand. But it is up to you as women to seal the deal by bringing *all* of your qualities to the table for us to benefit from them. It is not the man's fault that you have not devel-oped a sense of who you are so he can know what and who he is deal-ing with. So blaming us for an understanding you don't have about yourself is only going to have you at a disadvantage. But I have to be honest and say that some women are doomed from the start—because even though you have made it about you, you have made it about you in the wrong way.

CHAPTER 2

IT'S NOT ABOUT US (MEN)

During the time that my mom was alive, we would always have conversations about the way in which I would go about getting myself in a woman's life and what I was supposed to be doing to show a woman that I was the man that she had always been looking for. How was I going to show her that I would make all the difference in her life, if given the chance? How was I going to be able to meet her needs when society had already told her that she can do it herself? I really couldn't answer these questions at the time because like all the other men in our society no one had ever told me that…

"if I made it about women first, it will eventually become about me."

In the grand scheme of things, I didn't know what this meant as everything I had been taught since childhood, revolved around me proving myself to a woman. But then one day it hit me—what my mom had been trying to tell me all throughout the years. It was a humbling revelation, as I truly believed that I had been doing what I was supposed to be doing this whole time. But in reality, I wasn't. I was missing the *one* thing that could have made all the difference in most of my relationships, and probably some of yours as well. The thing I was missing was how important it was for a woman to tell me what she needed from me —*before* I could even begin to show to her my ability to do so. I was caught up in what I call the **"do process"** of being with a woman—instead of listening to what she desired in that **"do process."** And honestly, most men nowadays are caught up in that same mentality as well. For the most part, I agree with the mass population's belief that a man should prove to a woman that he deserves to be in her life; however, where I disagree is the way in which men have gone about it and the concepts on just how we are supposed to go about it.

I mean, how can any man prove that he is capable of doing the things that a woman needs him to do when most women don't even know what those things are? I find those questions to be very difficult for most women to answer from the start because most of you not only don't know what you need a man to do, but you don't even understand why it is so important for you to know what you need a man to do.

Well! I can't say that I entirely blame you more than I blame those people who continue to disregard or be ignorant to this concept. As we all know, a woman's way of doing things has taken over in our society. We have, for the most part, accepted the fact that the independent woman in America is here to stay. We have accepted the woman who says I have to be doing things to make my case that I am just as capable, or comparable as a man. But what if I told you that doing these things to make your case as a woman is the reason why man is looking down on you more than they ever have in our history? What if I told you that you are making a big mistake as women trying to get men to value your opinions and ideas through what you do as opposed to what you say? What would your response be?

Well! I can think of a couple of things some of you would say but I don't think that it would be appropriate to put in the book. But I am going to go there and say that most women are making a very big mistake acting as though men will take your opinions and ideas into account more through what you do than what you say. But he won't. Especially if your way of having things done for you puts him in the "helpmate" position more than the leading one! Most men try to hide the fact that they don't enjoy women bringing up the point that they have just as much ability to lead than they do. And no! Men don't feel this way because they feel that it will somehow make you seem masculine to them more than it makes them seem feminine to women. The reason why men feel this way is because they would rather women tell them how to be successful with them rather than exclude them and then have to take ridicule for not carrying out their natural position.

So many women have been sold on this new age way that as women you need to be doing in order to get the respect you deserve from a man. But you couldn't be more removed from the truth because no man respects a woman trying to sell herself on job related accolades and accomplishments. No man wants a woman making her case as the **"doer"** when he has been told all his life that he needs to be ready to do whatever it takes to be with you. Men have continuously approached you with their ears open and their eyes wide shut because you can't see the damage you are causing by not being the innovator of your own desires. They continuously approach you with that part of themselves that says "we need to be doing things for her,"—as you approach them with doing it yourselves. You have the opportunity as women to make your case that you understand the most important part of the **"do process"** between them and you. But you think the part that says this is the one that says you have to being doing it instead of getting a man to do it.

"You have made this about you in competition with a man, not realizing that you have made him incompetent to meeting your needs.

No one has told you that men think that the only reason why you're trying to make your case by doing it yourself is because you can't get a man to do it? The only reason you are paying your own bills, taking out the trash, taking your car to get an oil change, changing your tire when it gets flat or having some total stranger do it is because you have not the ability or the desire in your ability to get a man to do it? No one has told you that men think that the other reason you're doing it yourselves is because your girlfriends will talk bad about you if you let them do it? Not only that, but you don't even present men with the tone and temperament that will get a man to do anything for you because your girlfriends and society has told you that he will never value your opinions and ideas if you're only in the instruction part of the do process. He will never value your opinions and ideas if you let him do it and not show him that you can do it if you had to. But I am here to tell you that a man will never value your opinions and ideas as long as you continue to try and get those things through what you do as opposed to your ability to have him do it. A man will never value your opinions and ideas as long as you feel that you have to be at the forefront of the opinion or idea you're bringing to the table. A man will never value your opinions and ideas until you understand that….

"Your desire to get your needs met by a man has to be greater than his willingness to do it"

In order for a man to value the importance of your opinions and ideas from the start—you have to allow him to be in the **"do process"** of your desires. You have to allow him to be included, even though every one around you is telling you that he's not going to be up for the challenge. But he will be up for the challenge if you allow him to play his role in showing you. See, most women think that the doing part of the getting to know process is the most important part. But how can it be when no one is saying what needs to be done? I would describe it like a writer to a director. In the film industry, most people think that the most vital part of making a film is the director. It's just like being in the getting to know process where most people think that a man's position of doing is the most important part.

However, that's not true—because just like a writer, a woman wants to feel like her position is of value. That's why you have writers trying to be directors because they are not being giving the credit that they deserve for the most vital part of filmmaking. And that is… writing the screenplay. But without a screenplay or a script, there is really nothing there for a director to shoot or do! That same concept goes into the dynamic of a woman and a man. If a woman is not there to write the script on what a man needs to be directing in her life, he will never be given the grades he deserve for the academy award winning movie her family and friends have seen him direct in her life. So you tell me…. which person do you think is the most important person in the " do process" between men and women when they are getting to know each other?

"Is it the person who is saying what needs to be done or the person who is doing it?"

But what I am here to say is that if a man is successful in your life without playing his role in the "do process" between you and him, he will never value your opinions and ideas. He will never see you as the woman he was always looking for. Only the woman he was looking for at the moment. He will never see you as a commodity, but only as a woman who can be replaced at anytime! He will never see you as a treasure, only a trophy! Here it is—men are trying to be successful with you women through your ability to say what needs to be done. And yet, you continue to try and get those needs met by using the wrong approach to how you go about it. But I am here to say to you women that…

"A man will never do more to keep you, than he did to get you!"

The most tragic thing that most women do is think that they will be successful getting their needs met by men when you're not allowing men to be the doers in the do process of being with you. You have been told that you have to let a man do what a man is going to do, but if you're not saying what needs to be done, not only is he going to be unsuccessful in his attempt to show you that he is good listener—but he is going to feel like you're not good at telling him what needs to be done. In a sense, you are setting him up to feel like he can't trust you with telling him how he can be successful with you. That is when he will start to feel like he has to take it upon himself to adlib as to what he thinks you might want or need. You go along with his decision to be this way because you think that when you get in the relationship with him, he's going to give you the opportunity to show him that you have had the ability to tell him all along—but he's not because he doesn't TRUST you anymore than you have trusted his ability all this time! And once a man feels that he can't trust you with the most important part of satisfying your needs—that is when the problems will arise, especially when you get into the **"routine"** part of dealing with each other. As men, we know that it's not about us or it is not supposed to be about us from the start; but if we can't trust you with giving us a successful formula in being with you then we're going to start reverting back to the part of ourselves that says that we can fix it. That we can be the difference between you and us being successful in making your case to a society and the people around you who have set the two of us up to fail on their way of doing things.

But that's where I come in to say that you will never be successful with men when your opinions and desires are being taking for granted and out of context. You will never be successful with men as long as you continue to disregard the importance of understanding that your word is bond—and not his from the start. You will never be successful with men as long as you continue to feel like you can't trust them with your opinions and desires, and are willing to believe that men *are* ready and willing participants. You will never be successful with men as long as you continue to believe that it is up to men to make a case that they are able instead of you making sure that a man can be successful in making his case that they are able. Looking at television and listening to the radio, one of the things that have been lost in translation is that most women are making it about them but in the wrong way.

From shows such as *The Bachelor, Tough LOVE and even, Millionaire Matchmaking* "one of the things that I found that was truly being overlooked is the way in which the men on those shows were making things all about women. In almost every episode, the women on those shows were being told to let the men show them that they can be the men that you have been always looking for instead of being told that as women they have to be ready to make sure that these men were capable of being what they were always looking for. Yes! You may know that a man can meet some of your wants by his own interpretation of things. However, that does not mean that he can meet your needs or even have any desire to do so for the long term. And just because he can make a few of your so called fairytale dreams come true, doesn't mean that when reality sets in that he will be ready to accept the part of you that needs more out of him. So it's up to me to tell you that….

"There is absolutely no way that a man will ever be able to meet your needs through his way of doing things."

He may be able to meet your wants! But in order for him to be a complete man in your life you have to be able to tell him what you need from him—and not merely settle for what he is willing to give you. There are but a few men on planet earth who are truly capable of meeting a woman's wants. Let alone her needs! Especially in this day and age when love is not the most important component any-more! As a woman, you have to know that you will not be successful in getting the best out of a man's ability when you're not presenting them with the necessary desires that will stand up against ridicule, opinions and skepticism. The only reason why society, your family and your girlfriends have an argument about your future mate is because they have had an argument about your ability to show a man how to be successful in your life. They have known you all of your life, and nothing that you say to them is going to get them to believe you until you start saying these things to the man in your life to make a case with them outside of it. Because in the end…

"You will never be able to make your case with them until you are able to make your case with him."

Men think that the people in your life are talking about them when they are really talking about your inability to tell them what needs to be done, while you insist upon being an "independent woman." You don't see that your family and friends have made it all about you and are not trying to help you realize it because it gives them the right to question you and your desires. They don't even have the ability to help you in your quest to get your needs met, but yet they want to question the way in which you go about it. Your cry out for society's help and assistance has fallen on deaf ears, because nothing about their life masked yours, if you let society tell it. You are on your own! Never once did any of the people around you tell you that it was your ability to tell him what needed to be done that was in question more than his ability to do it.

Now, I will play devil's advocate and say that there are women who feel that they have a case when talking about man's inability to meet their needs in the **"do process"** of being with them. That maybe it was the man who was just unable to interpret what those needs were. Well…. let me be frank in saying this. A man will always be able to meet your needs when you are clear as to what those needs are—especially in the **"getting to know"** process because being unsuccessful in a position where he knows that he is not in control will never allow him the right to be in a position of receiving and/or benefiting. He will never be in a position where you, as a woman, will or should ever give him the right to be anything to you beyond a distant memory. And you should not be allowing the people in your life to tell you otherwise.

Like I said earlier, your girlfriends will make it seem like they are talking about the guy who is trying to make it about you—rather than being honest in saying that they are using him as the scapegoat to talk about your inabilities. Man has never been unsuccessful in accomplishing the things that have been made extremely clear for him to do or be about, because he knows that he can't win without your interpretation or desire. He will never fail at those things if he doesn't have to go on an educated guess of how he goes about getting it done. So I am here to tell you that if you as women don't start telling men about your desires and letting him meet them instead of doing them yourselves…

"you will always have problems with men."

Here it is! Men are trying to make it all about you. But you're in the way of allowing him to show you what you have always been worth. However, because you can't see it, your friends can't see it, your mom can't see it and all the other people whose judgment you trust—you stop the man in your life from being the equalizer in the game of "cat and mouse" that you and all of your co-conspirators have brought to the table. The people in your life feel that their opinion of your life matters more than your desires to have one. So what you think about yourself and how you get your needs met doesn't matter.

You have allowed them to be part of every bad choice and decision you have made for so long, that they only see you as a willing participant in their crusade to ruin another potential mate for you. In short, your attitude was that you had to keep the part about getting your needs met secret from them because they would have something negative to say about it. But then you will confide in them when it doesn't work out with Mr. Right! And you wonder why your abilities are always in question. You think that he is supposed to create his own expectations to live by. But it is not **TRUE!** As a woman, you are the most important element in the **"do process"** between you and a man.

"It is not his job to create your expectations of him…it's *your* job to do that." "

Some of you have even convinced yourselves, or have allowed society to convince you—that you don't have the ability to get your needs met unless you're doing it yourselves. And when most men don't automatically do it—you revert back to blaming them for the fact that you didn't get what you deserved. But if you were playing your role in getting what you deserved— you wouldn't have to blame anyone. So often I am faced with those women who tell me that the reason men get blamed for not being successful at meeting their needs is because they feel that if a man wants to meet their needs that he should just do it and then I will tell him later what I like and what I don't like. But what I would like to know is when has a man ever gone on his own decision making process to make up a woman's mind for her? What man would ever do that? What man would take a chance on failing by insisting upon doing things his way and not waiting for a woman to tell him? He knows that….

"It is a one way street… hopefully leading to a two way street"

And I recommend that you women start seeing it this way. You should be prepared to let everyone know that it is and should be about you from the start. In addition, you should be further prepared to let everyone know that you have the ability to tell a man how you want things done. You need to be ready to fight for your right to have a man do good by you and treat you well. You need to be ready to motivate, encourage and inspire a man to do those things so that he can validate your reasons for taking a chance on him. But most of all…you need to be ready to be the woman who says you are going to create the expectations for him to fulfill.

Honestly, there's nothing more frustrating than trying to meet a woman's needs who has no ability to tell me what they are. There is nothing more ignorant than a woman who says that she wants a real man and when one presents himself, she has no clue as to what she needs "Mr. Real Man" to do. There is nothing more confusing than a woman who claims to hate men for not making it about her, but then is always being negative when she is around men and makes it official that it will never be that way. There is nothing sadder than a woman who has the ability to get her needs met, but is letting the people around her stop her from doing so because their desires mean more to her than her own. However, there is nothing more tragic than a woman who never makes a decision on one man because she's scared she is going to ruin the possibility of getting her needs met by all the other men she has given free reign in her life.

I brought up these women to say this: A man's chance to make the point that he is capable of meeting your needs does not come from his way of doing things. It comes from *your* way of saying what needs to be done. Therefore, taking any responsibility for interpreting the way in which a woman gets her needs met from the start is not something that he should do. There is no way that he should allow you to sit back while he takes a beating he could have avoided. As a man, he wants to help defend your reasons for taking a chance on him. He wants your reasons to be validated by what he does—and not what *you* do! But he cannot accomplish those things successfully, if what is being said *to* him and *about* him is in direct conflict with what is being expected *from* him.

I always knew that I was going to be the kind of man who would not only defend my girl's reasons for taking a chance on me, but also one who would validate those reasons according to what I did. I also knew that I would never be able to defend her reasons for taking a chance on me if I allowed her to be in the way of that process. Your family and friends don't understand that you like him for being him. They don't understand that you genuinely love him for no reason beyond the conventional guy you've gone out with. That's why you have to understand that in order for the people in your life not to have an argument, you have to be willing to be at the forefront of the "do process" between you and the man you decided to take a chance on. You have to be willing to say as a woman that….

"I am going to be the reason for a man being successful with me, so he will be able to defend and validate my reasons for taking a chance on him. "

And if you're not ready to do your part to insure that it is going to be about you, then don't be angry when it's not about you. If you're not going to do your part to insure that things go your way, then don't be mad when you don't get the results that you believe you deserve. If you're not going to do your part to insure that he is going to make your case for you by what he does, then don't be mad when you're met with a host of complaints and negative talk about him. Most people would look at your situation and say that birds of a feather usually flock together. But that's really not the case because he is not really bringing on this ridicule with what he is doing more than you are bringing it on with what you are saying needs to be done. He couldn't be more confused with this whole situation as he tries to incorporate his way of doing things and combine it with your way of having it done. Even when he has convinced you that he is capable of meeting your needs, you're not really the person that he is worried about convincing. It is the people that *you* confided in who said he had no chance with you—because they already knew that your way of doing things sets men up to fail every time.

They look at you and they think that they will give you a pass because he should know better than to take a chance on a woman like you because they know that you don't see any worth in yourself. So asking this man to defend his reasons for being chosen by you is a joke to them. That is the very reason that blaming you for something that you were incapable of accomplishing from the start—simply doesn't make sense. Man is once again taking the blame for not only his inability to defend your reasons for taking a chance on him, but his inability to figure out how to get you to tell him what your needs are as well. But it's not about men, even though you seem to be okay with that. To be honest… we don't even expect to be given such a gift from the start. And those men who have made it all about themselves at the start will never make it about you in the relationship because like I said earlier in the chapter…

"A man will never do more to keep you than he did to get you."

This is what you should be thinking about when you first meet a man. Is he willing to make it all about me before I decide to make it about him? Is he willing to defend and validate my reasons for taking a chance on him? Or is he going to be one of those kind of men who think that his way of doing things takes precedence over my way of wanting them done? As a woman, you should be encouraged and motivated to get a man to see things your way. It should make you feel good that man is willing to take a chance on showing you that it could be about you for a long time. It should also make you feel good to know that someone is willing to validate your reasons for taking a chance on them. And if done right, you may have the man that you have said all of your life that you were looking for!

That's what every man has been looking for—a woman who respected herself enough to make it about herself from the start. This kind of woman is special. She is the kind of woman that gets a man excited about carrying out his position in her life! She is the kind of woman who could ruin the negativities of a man and replace it with a chivalrous heart. What kind of woman are you? Are you the kind who likes people talking about your inability to get to the very core of a man? Or are you the kind of woman who looks forward to bringing out the potential in a man? Are you the kind of woman that men run from? Or are you the kind of woman that a man can't wait to move forward with? Are you the kind of woman who sees her future being with a loving, supportive man or are you the kind of woman who dwells on the past? This is the kind of woman you should be aspiring to be. A motivator of men! And men, we are no different! We need to start telling these women that we are ready to carry out our positions in their lives and trust that we will get it done.

Even the independent woman would take a backseat to a man and let him do all the things she claims makes her an independent woman, if she knew that she could trust a man's ability to make the case for her with her pitty party of five. Society has told her lies about men, which has resulted in her being in a position that she never intended to be in. But she can't help herself because men have not made it about her in a long time. We have not fought for them. We have not even tried. What's truly sad is that we both claim to want the same thing. Men claim that they want to be the men that you've always been looking for. And women claim that they want to be the women that you've always been looking for—and yet we both have sat back and let those people who have no clue on what our desires are tell us that in order to achieve the ultimate goal we have to take on a role never intended for anyone of us to be in. "You're going to be a better woman if you take away man's ability to make the case for you. And you're going to be a better man if you allow her to take away your ability to make the case for her." And ultimately, society will praise you for finally seeing things their way. But they won't praise you. However, they will pat themselves on the back because they were right about the fact that there is no possible way that you as a woman will ever be able to get a man to defend or validate your reasons for taking a chance on him because you won't tell him what he needs to be doing in order to do so. It's funny how….

"You have catered to society's way of talking bad about you."

You have fed into your own demise. Like I said, they have known you for quite a while now. And even though they know that if you ever came to your senses and realized that you have been this way, they can always make their case by saying that you never fought back or complained. So how did they know how you really felt when you never said anything? How did they know that you always knew that you could get a man to make things about you when nothing gave them the indication that you could do so? And if you could—why didn't you make your case sooner? You have had more than enough time and chances! You have had more than enough potentials and possibilities. But how can you take away ridicule and complaint if you're not good at your job so that the man you choose can be good at his?

You're just now realizing that you had it all WRONG! But you didn't have it all wrong. They did! Society was feeding a part of you that never existed and not feeding the part of you that did. Society was beating down your ability to get a man to make it about you because no one had told them that the most important position to be played was the person saying what needed to be done and not the person doing it. So how could they tell you about something they've had no clue in knowing? How could they help you see the truth about yourself when they have struggled to see the truth about themselves? You should be encouraged to know that you have had this ability all of your life. It is not about men from the start. It never WAS! As women, most of you even have the feeling that you don't care how it becomes about you. As long as it becomes that way! But I am here to tell you that in a perfect world that would be nice. But a real man knows that his true success is wrapped up in your ability to tell him how things are done and not his. He knows that his true success is wrapped up in his ability to let you know that he values your opinions and ideas more than his own. He knows that his true success is wrapped up in being able to follow the rules more than create them. There is an old saying that......

"a happy wife brings on a happy life"

But I would go a step further in saying that the only way they got to that point was through her ability to make it about herself at the start and not allowing a man to give her less than she was willing to say she needed in order to get to that point. When I look at most of the relationships that are not working or have not worked today, I attribute the start as the reason why they have failed. I can assure you that many women did not successfully carry out their ability to get a man to make it about them.

The world is changing before our eyes, however, that doesn't mean that you have to change along with it. That doesn't mean that you have to be brainwashed into thinking that your success with a man or a woman is ever going to come from a society that is all about their interpretation of your life and not your own. You don't have to be brainwashed into thinking that in order to fit in you have to allow society to make it about themselves while stopping you from getting a man to help defend and validate your reasons for taking a chance on him. Men are in your CORNER! They just need you to quit throwing jabs and start hitting your family and friends with some real blows as they are pulling punches with you. As long as you continue to allow the people around you to make it about them—thus preventing the man in your life from validating his reasons for being chosen by you, they will always have an ARGUMENT!

"Be the SAYER and not the DOER!"

Be the woman who truly understands that in order for you to be okay in your relationship—you have to be open to a man making things easier for you. And what better way to start then by seeing that you have the ability to tell a man what needs to be done and trusting that he will get it done. Otherwise, see him for what he is and move on so you can see if the next man is up for making it about you. You have to get it through your head that some men don't even know that their true success is wrapped up in their ability to make it about you first. And if he is not a man who knows this just yet, don't be mad at him—but don't be anything else either. Let the next woman try and navigate him to that place of understanding this concept. You're looking for a real man. If there is one thing that I would want you to take away from this book it would be this:

"*men care more about what you say than what you do.*"

And until our society start taking more stock in what is being said than what is being done, women will always have a problem seeing that their position is the most important position of all. You will always struggle with your ability to get a man to take on his role because you think that his role is the most important role and you don't like feeling like you're taking a backseat to it. You will always struggle with your position in saying what needs to be done because you don't want to take responsibility for what you think is the least important position. But it isn't! And never was…. A man knows that he can be successful with you and for you without a doubt! But it's going to take you women out there playing your role to get him to that point. Sitting back and waiting for him to meet your needs without the words he needs to do so—is not a good idea by any stretch of the imagination. So you better start taking the initiative and tell a man how you want things done.

No one ever said that it was going to be easy. No one ever said that it was going to be something that every man that comes into your life is willing to do. What I am saying is that there is going to come a time in your life where you are going to be face-to- face with the man you have always wanted. Not being ready to help him be successful is only going to have you failing at proving your point that you are ready for the chance of a lifetime. But now that you know that a man's success is based on your ability to tell him what to do, there is a certain attitude that comes with this approach.

CHAPTER 3

"Right Approach, Wrong Attitude"

Every now and again during the "meet and greet process," I will find a man and a woman who understand the equation of *God, man* and *woman*—and how this positioning plays a vital role in both sexes getting their needs met. However, what often happens is that we have to fight off a certain attitude in order for it to work. When I think about what attitude we have to fight off in order for things to work, the word **"sense of entitlement"** comes to mind. We have a sense of entitlement attitude that has us thinking that something or someone is owed to us. From the moment we began tipping the waitress at the coffee shop for pouring our coffee, or tipping the cashier for ringing us up for an overpriced carwash, or having people super size us at the fast food place, we have laid the groundwork for people to take us for granted and/or get more than they deserved. But the question I would like to ask is…

"Who are we to expect more out of a person when we are giving off an attitude that we don't truly deserve it?"

We have created this above and beyond attitude that has created the basis for the "little things" to go unappreciated. On one end we are giving people above and beyond credit for doing exactly what they already are being given credit for doing. And yet, not giving credit to those people who are doing things that deserve an honorable mention. I was always told that you get what you pay for. But as time has gone on it seems as though just giving someone credit for what they have done is not enough.

Usually when you give someone something, whether its credit, attention or anything for that matter, more than likely you're going to expect something in return— when your main focus should be on pleasing that person beyond your own desires. What you think you deserve should not be measured in what someone is willing to give you—more than what God is willing to bless you with. That is why I always make it my business to tell people that if they want to do something for me, to do it unconditionally because I can't give them a better return on that investment more than God. We have become a society that either *needs* to be reciprocated for things we didn't do—or we expect "an above and beyond" return for the things that we have done.

Oftentimes, in the getting to know process—you're going to come across people who claim to be set in their ways and really believe that they don't need to change certain things about themselves or their situation in order to get what they want. Denial has become the drug of choice for many adults—who feel that *eventually* their attitude and approach is going to render a better result. But as the old saying goes…

"If you keep coming with the same ole' approach and attitude… you're going to keep getting the same 'ole result."

I have seen this concept played out one time too many in the minds and hearts of human beings who truly believe that someone or something is going to eventually like and accept the way things are. So the question now becomes more about a person's ability to wait for the one person who can accept the way things are—rather than change the way things are and give themselves more options. Even though their attitude should be that of a person who is looking for one mate to accept them for who they are—that doesn't mean ruin or rule out all the other possibilities by being set in those ways.

It's like a fishermen who cast a small net and expects to catch a *lot* of fish. He is only limiting the possibility of catching as many fish as possible. Sadly, at times this is how we behave as men and women! We have a tendency to limit ourselves by casting a "small part" of ourselves to the world. Of course you may have to throw back a few men and women for them to fully develop as a "potential catch," but at least you have cast a wide enough net to give yourself plenty of potentials and/or opportunities.

One of the things I always hear women saying is if somebody doesn't like them for who they are—they really don't care because they're not going to change. Their attitude has told them that there is no need for change. And so! They go on not only "ruining the possibility of many" with this attitude but "ruining the potentials" of one because the many that didn't oblige have created a negative "sense of entitlement attitude" in you—which now has your attitude turning off the one person who was interested in finding out more about you. Even after I have seen this attitude in someone as I observe their situation and let them know that this is going, do they still carry on as if nothing is wrong. And so! What I have learned in this instance is that…

"Most women would rather be comfortable in being wrong than being uncomfortable in being right."

Some women would rather accept the way things are because they don't know anything else beyond sabotaging their own worth. That's why they go on ruining the potentials of one after the other men wanted no part in dealing with them. Those women couldn't censor their attitudes that would have and could have given them better experiences leading up to Mr. Right. I can speak for most men when I say that the most important thing to a man when dealing with a woman is a woman's tone and temperament when it is being gentle and pleasing. So I must go out on a limb and tell women that it is not the demands from you that bother us as men. It is the sense of entitlement attitude that you present us with that bother us. But to me, the days of women being gentle and pleasing are over because women feel that the days of needing a man the way my mom and grandmother did are no larger an important part of a woman's makeup.

The attitude that women can "make it without a man" has definitely presented itself in the last twenty years. It has become a very commonplace thing for me to hear women saying this. But the one thing I've noticed is that I only hear the single women saying these things and accepting them for what they are. For those women who are truly looking for a mate, I don't know how you have allowed the single and the naïve to speak on your behalf as to how you go about getting our needs met and the tone and temperament in which you do it. And contrary to belief…. no man is looking for a woman with an *attitude problem*. The majority of men don't even like to be around women who present themselves in that way. But if you let society tell it man seems to resonate to the BITCHY woman!

"Yeah… if he wants an excuse not to act right or not feel bad about acting right."

When I think about the women of today, the word strong seems to come to mind—if only for the sake of argument which doesn't seem to set well with me and some of my male counterparts who feel that we don't see or think of women in this way because it gives off a masculine interpretation that doesn't give us an image that attracts us to you. And though time after time when women have clarified for me what they have meant by using this phrase—it still doesn't make me feel much for taking on a role that is going to give us the best chance to succeed. It also doesn't seem like it's something women are going to be willing to take part in anyway! So I asked myself, "Why bother with taking on a position in a woman's life that she is not going to be proud and/or appreciative of? Why put myself in a position to be taken for granted by someone who has no desire to acknowledge my making things easier for her?"

From the moment I started dating online, I would say that almost every profile I have read by a woman—she described herself as a "strong" woman or an "independent" woman—which I have already learned doesn't sit well with the real man in America. I definitely think that one of the reasons for the confusion is that we as men never heard our mothers and grandmothers saying that they were strong women and/or independent women. And secondly, the word strong used to be the way we describe men back then. So now that most women have taken over this word or the interpretation of this word, how do we as men describe ourselves these days without making it seem like we are taking a backseat to women? Because all it makes me feel like is that you're claiming to…

"Act like a woman while thinking like a man."

And for the records, ladies! If you hear a man say out loud or writing on his internet profile that he's looking for a strong woman or an independent woman, he is telling you that he is looking for an excuse not to be the man that you're going to need in your life for the long haul. So if you want to be with a man like that—then do me and all of mankind a favor and don't complain when his true colors come to the table. Now for the sake of argument, I will play devil's advocate and say that I understand women coming at men with the attitude that you have to be strong in order to make it in this world today. But I am here to tell you that if you approach every man with this attitude— you are not going to get your needs met. We as men never had to clarify our reasons for using the word "strong". So we don't understand why most women would use a word to describe yourselves and then have to come with an explanation to validate your reason for using it. I don't understand this reasoning! I mean…. "Where did this attitude come from?"

Oftentimes, I will ask a woman where this attitude of not allowing men to make things easier for them comes from—and I am usually told that they were taught this by their parents. But I have to admit that it left me confused that a mom and a dad who didn't grow in an era where women would ever say these things is now teaching their children the opposite of how they were raised. I would find it to be extremely ignorant that a woman who never degraded men or her position with one, is now teaching her daughter to have this attitude. But okay …if you say so! I just have a hard time believing that a woman who has been married to the same man for thirty years, and he's been a stand-up guy all of her life—is now telling her daughter that she should be approaching men in a different manner than she did with her own husband.

Unfortunately, many women are not alone in this attitude even if you are in the approach that I am about to bring to your attention. Unlike most of my male counterparts, I love older women. To be honest with you, I have become the butt of many jokes by my friends who joke that I won't date a woman unless she smells like Efferdent or Polygrip! But I will go out a limb and say that there is nothing more beautiful than an older woman—at least not to me! So what I'm about to say is not only crazy, but tragic. And that is these older women that think that having the same attitude and approach that the younger women have is going to get them anywhere with men. This is the most tragic thing that I have seen since television and magazines have taken it upon themselves to tell women that looking young, coincides with acting young. But I am here to tell you that it does no such thing. And I know that most of you women are going to hate to read this. But I don't know how to tell you any other way without you getting an attitude anyway. So I'm going to tell you that…..

"there is nothing more unattractive than an older woman with an attitude problem."

And you know who you are! The one who is at the nightclub with your daughter acting as though you never had a chance to shine because you got married too young and now it's your time to stand out. Or the woman who is still dressing provocatively when your body is not permitting that to happen. News flash! You had your opportunity to sell a man on those things when you were young, but you're not young anymore! And even though you are able to cheat age, if only for a little while, doesn't mean that you are benefiting from the way you look now more than you did when you were young. And if your friends or family don't have the guts to tell you that you are making a fool of yourself, let me be the first to tell you that...

"You're making a fool out of yourself"

Now, I understand that the magazines have you believing that 40 is the new 30. That 50 is the new 40. But what the magazines forgot to tell you is that to a man 40 is still 40! And 50 is really being 60 when you're carrying the attitude of a 24-year-old. Acting this way *doesn't* get the guy. It only gets the guy to ignore you and think of you as a woman with no self control. And once again, I know what the argument is going to be for those of you in America who feel as though your days are just beginning. That you like yourself more at 40 and 50 because you're not the woman questioning who you are and how you're supposed to act around men. I understand that you're not the woman who is questioning your sexuality anymore and how society has stopped you from really seeing the truth about yourself. That you're a woman and you feel more alive than ever and there is still a great possibility of finding love out there for you.

Well, I am here to tell you that those things are not out there for a woman with an attitude problem. And definitely not for a woman that thinks that age is just a number, while having an attitude problem. It may be just a number to you but to a man it's a reality. A reality that makes him feel like in order to stay young, that he has to look at the daughter more than the mother—who is presenting him with the daughter's attitude. He may find that attitude "cute" in the daughter—but not in you as her mother. Sadly, most women who have read those magazines and listened to society's interpretations of beauty—have fallen into the trap of not only looking young, but acting young as well. Unfortunately, acting like a 24 year old while being a woman that is mature in age, has an ignorance to it that takes away the soul essence of growing old because as we get older we don't want to be seen as such—even if we feel that way.

When I was dating online, it fascinated me how so many women lied about their age, in order to snag a younger man. And their excuse for this was… "Men my age look more like my father than a potential mate." But if you think about it, it doesn't leave the older men with many options—other than the one where he tries to "buy" his way into a young woman's life. Why do you think we have such a contrast in our society? Because no one has the attitude of **"let's grow old together"** anymore! That sense of entitlement attitude— that *I am going to get what I want even if I have to buy it* has things more screwed up than ever.

But I am here to tell you that if you have this attitude it will ruin your approach every time. You may even have the best of intentions, but simply not realize that your attitude is what's stopping you from having someone appreciate you for really being something special. And I do understand that, as a woman, selling men on who you are as an older woman is going to be a lot harder than selling them on what you were as a young hottie. So as a young woman, you need to take advantage of the youth you possess, because it's going to be hard to convince a man of who you are when you get older. Especially if you're one of those women with the attitude, that you can take away a man's position to make a case for your own. As an older woman, you should be selling a man from the inside, out! Not the outside, in because…

"What you were as a young woman was giving you the opportunity to sell him on who you are now as an older one."

I have even had to bring these findings up to the women in my life where it seems that the younger women are trying to sell men on their accomplishments, their intellect, their job and all the other things that man is not impressed with. And the older women are trying to sell men on their sex appeal, looks and all the things you are doing to stay young. But what man is really impressed with is the glow you have from being in love with life and your desire for a man. A man is impressed with the way you walk into a room with a humble, yet eloquent confidence.

However, a man is not impressed by the woman coming through the door like a **"perfect storm"** making sure she leaves nothing in her path but chaos and destruction. You have even given this impression to those who have no motivation one way or the other about you because they could care less. But because you were so overwhelming in your attempt to be seen and heard, it was hard for them to overlook you. And for as much as you think we do as men... we do not want a woman who is an open book. I'm talking about a woman whose been revealed to everyone. In such a case, there's "nothing new under the sun" to share with family and friends— because they already know your entire history. You're not a mystery! To them, you're just MISERY!

There are so many women that grade themselves by the woman who just came in through the front door at the restaurant, or by the woman in the bathroom, or the woman in the party who seems to be getting all of the attention! But yet! You don't know that it was her "womanly qualities" that got her that attention and not all of the accolades and accomplishments she could muster up. Men are more concerned with your womanly qualities more than anything else that you could bring to the table. And if you don't have a clue of what I am talking about as far as womanly qualities then I suggest you find a woman in your life where her approach has worked with men and figure out what you're doing wrong. Men want to know if they are going to need sunglasses because you came into the room like a bright light, or if they are going to need insurance for the mess you're going to create. And just for the record, ladies!

"Men want to know about your sex appeal before your intellect appeal."

That doesn't mean that you have to tear down his desire to be chivalrous because you can't seem to get beyond the fact that he wants to appreciate your beauty more than your work ethic and your accomplishments. I mean… you should be happy that you still make a man excited when being around you. You should be appreciative that a man still goes out of his way to acknowledge you for the fact that you have kept yourself together and not let yourself go. **Not a woman with an attitude who thinks and feels that every time a man compliments you, he is only interested in the physical part of you more than the intellectual part of you.** In fact, you should be worried if a man *doesn't* want to be intimate with you, because how else will you be given the opportunity to show him that you are more than that? Ladies, it's not our being intimate with you that keep things interesting to us—it's your sex appeal because….

"There is nothing about you that men want more than you."

So quit allowing your girlfriends, family members and society in general to sell you on how men think and feel. Create your own experience and stop being influenced by the experience of others. Do not carry your sister's burdens with men into your life. Be the woman you set out to be!

There is nothing more rewarding than a woman being willing in spirit and mind. There is nothing more beautifully displayed than a woman who knows that she doesn't have to sell herself to a man with an attitude that doesn't reflect the approach. Coming at man with a sense of entitlement attitude that *you're not going to be appreciative of him* making things easier for you is not going to get your needs met. Now I know most women have seen or heard, or even experienced the right approach with a man before and it may not have worked out for you. But that still doesn't give you the right to think that the next man should have to fight through an attitude created by the guy you just got rid of. Because contrary to what you believe…

"A man will never carry the burden of a "history" that he didn't create."

He will never take an emotional and mental beating from you that he didn't cause. So what is the point that you are making when you are stopping a man from meeting your needs and then being mad when he doesn't? What is the point you are trying to make when a man is trying to show you that you are worth everything he is trying to do for you, but you can't even appreciate it? And why do some of you women think that men should take this laying down? I'm sure that I can speak for a lot of men when I say that men are tired of not only being faced with this attitude that we have to fight through your experiences and your previous relationship to please you, but being considered "mean" or "cruel" the minute we don't accept this atti- tude as such.

    This has been a tactic that most women have gotten away with. And you wonder why men are no longer going out of their way to please women. Did it ever occur to you that you have created this lack of desire in men? Did it ever occur to you that men have become just as tired of the beating they have taken just trying to be a team player? Many of you are asking yourselves right now how any man can say what I am saying. But it's about time women heard the hard- core truth about why men have no desire anymore! Most women call it laziness! But it's not laziness. It is a lack of desire that he has. "So why is it a lack of desire, Tonee?" Well, there are a lot of women who feel that love will never exist for them anyway. So you go into the getting to know process with the attitude that….

"If it happens, it happens! And if it doesn't! Well… I didn't think that it would anyway."

I mean…. why should any man show you something that you never deemed as possible? You can't see the big picture! So why should he start drawing? He feels the same way that every man has felt dealing with you. That he has no business putting himself out there for a woman with an unbelieving heart anyway! He has told himself that there is definitely no room for him to convince you to accept what you already do not believe in. You have even gone as far as to tell him about all the other men you sabotaged on your continuous crusade of being what you despised in other people. You have become this person who thinks that everyone is trying to take you for a ride, all the while you have been taking men on the ride of their lives. Your defense has been that all these men don't know you—and that may very well be true—but what never occurred to you is that they don't care to know you because...

"They know that they are going to have to use up the energy in who they are, just to get you to see *yourself*."

Which by the way they are not interested in doing. This whole concept of being the "future boyfriend" all the while playing counselor, minister and therapist just doesn't appeal to their way of doing things. Even if they are getting their degree in these fields, the last thing they want to do, is to find themselves sleeping with the enemy and/or a future patient. A man may see your beauty and tell himself that he can overlook a few things that have his red flags waving. But then he catches himself because he knows that in the long run that won't keep him from being drained by the inevitable. And that is— you are not a woman who is going to be satisfied unless you're making things more difficult. But I am here to tell you that...

"A man will be helpless and no good to you when you keep him dwelling on the things he can't help you with—as opposed to the things that he can."

Even as most of you women read about yourselves in this book, you keep telling yourselves that me and every other man in America has no idea what we're talking about; therefore, you're going to keep going with your attitude because there's no way that you can't convince one man to take a chance on meeting your needs. Well! If he likes punishment, you will. But if he is anything like I know a man to be, you will definitely be a mute point to him in a couple of weeks.

Some of you women have created the equation for not only you to live by in your life, but for the men you are choosing as well. Men have definitely taken you at your word that you are going to make it as difficult as possible for him to meet your needs! And even though he hasn't let you in on his plans to leave you "high and dry" because of that attitude, he can't wait for you to give him that ultimate excuse to be done with you.

That's why men love women with **ATTITUDES**! Because there is always a way out whenever he feels like the situation has gotten out of hand and repetitive. Even for the most patient of men. Other than belief, I don't think that there is anything that could ruin the possibilities of something more than attitude. It will have the most patient men understanding why no one wants to have anything to do with you. So who are you to think that someone will overlook your attitude to try and please you? I have been told by some women that men find it to be cute that they have a bit of an attitude.

Well, here's a news flash for those of you who think that men feel that having a little bit of an attitude is "cute." If you want a man who will be looking for a way out of his responsibilities with you, all you have to do is to continue showing him that you have an "attitude problem" and I promise you it will be over before it has even begun. I don't know who came up with this concept that men think having a little bit of attitude is cute, anyway! And I know what the next argument is going to be with some women. What Tonee? I know you're not asking me to just bow down to a man? Well! If that's what you think I have been telling you all this time, then maybe this whole dating thing is not for you. What I am saying is that you don't need to overwhelm a man who is ready to meet your needs with the attitude of the one who wasn't. And those women who are getting their needs met by the men in their lives are not bowing down to men.

"They are bowing down to their DESIRES."

You don't need to bring your frustrations from your previous relationship to the table with the next guy to show that you're not going to put up with the negative things you dealt with before him. You don't need to break down every bad experience to every man for them to get what you're trying to say. We get it! We're just trying to get you to understand that we get it. Here it is...

"We as men have been trying to meet your needs through what you claim you want. But you keep trying to get every man to meet your needs through what you claim you don't want."

Ultimately, men are trying to meet your needs. And yet! Most of you won't even lose the attitude to present us with a better motivation and desire. You don't understand that men are not going to be motivated to do the things that are going to show you that he deserves an honorable mention and chance to be with you if he knows that your attitude is going to get in the way. And I encourage you men out there in society to get a backbone about yourselves and start singing the same tune.

Challenge a woman to be appreciative more than angry. Challenge her to be elegant more than trashy. Challenge her to see that you have been ready since day one to show her that with her support you can be the man she has always been looking for. It is the only way that you're going to get the respect you deserve from a woman. As a man, you have to have the same **"I'm not willing to settle"** mentality that they have when dealing with you. I know that for the most part there are some women who have somewhat of a sense of how to approach the "getting to know process with men.

But it seems like we have always gone on the "minority" report to give us the "majority' s perception."

We have always gone on people's opinions that matter the least to give the perspective of those people who desires that matters the most. But for the time being, I guess I am going to enjoy being on the men's side of the fence. It's definitely not something that we have taken a part in creating, this new aged way of thinking. And I am sure that I speak for a lot of men who feel this way as well. Even though man's position seems to be lost in translation at the current time doesn't mean that we're lost for good. It just means that we need to find ourselves. And there is nothing that is going to help our cause more than to say to women in general—lose the attitude so that I don't have an excuse not to consider you or your desires the way that I was taught. Men have just as much right as you not to deal with a woman taking him for granted and expecting anything beyond **"I'll see you later"** because at the end of the day, he has to look himself in the mirror and know that he is being the best that he can be for you as a man.

What most women don't understand is that when a man feels like he is not getting the respect he deserves or will never get the respect he deserves for trying to meet your needs, **"shame"** will set in. Even if you are sleeping with him and allowing him to spend time with you! He is not looking for better because he doesn't want to be with you. He is looking for better because you have never really appreciated the consistency he has brought to your doorstep. You have never really appreciated the stability that he has brought to your life. You have never given him the credit for how easy he has made things in the last two months being with you. You think that you are rewarding him with the very thing you thought that he was after in the first place. "Sex"! But he wasn't after sex! He was after something that the sexual or physical could never give him. He was after something that money couldn't buy. He was after something that none of his friends could give him. He was after your acknowledgement of his position in your life. He was after your feeding his ego. He was after your tone and temperament that brings on a joyful noise to his ears. He was after "you".

But you just couldn't see what he was really after. And now the "shame" is so great that he has no other choice but to free himself from your life. Some of you don't realize that your attitude is taking away a man's desire to be there for you. You don't realize that every time a man looks at you, he sees you as the reminder that he has taken a backseat to your so-called independence and that just does not work for him and his psychological approach as a man. And you're not going to get that out of any man if every time one of us come at you with our approach, the first thing that you present us with is your **"attitude"** that you are no more interested in their position in your lives more than you are with your position in ours! There doesn't always have to be a benefit for you to use common courtesy towards men. And with that being said:

"If you keep coming at men with the wrong attitude, you are leaving them with no other option but to come at you with the wrong approach."

Having the wrong attitude will not convince a man that he needs to go any further with you. If anything, having the wrong attitude is only going to further his intentions and desires to get his needs met because he knows that he's not going to be around you that long. You accuse him of not having the right motives from the start because he has no more desire to continue trying to get in your world or be in your world the way you see fit. I have experienced these kinds of accusations in my own dealings with women who refuse to see that they were the ones that were ruining the "getting to know" process between us and not me. I mean….. Why should I or any other man deal with any woman blaming us for an approach we have no control over or didn't create in you in the first place? Here we are trying to show women that we are capable of sustaining our positions in your lives and you're making it hard for us to do. But it is true….

A man will sustain his position with you as long as he knows that you will always let him know how much you are pleased with his primary position of making things easier for you. And if you're not a woman that has the ability or the desire to inspire, encourage or motivate a man to carry out this approach, then don't be mad when he doesn't do it. I have seen the right attitude in women who don't want a man to make things easier for them. And I have seen the wrong attitude in women who actually want a man to make things easier for them. Nothing is more confusing for a man because we know that women for the most part are not trying to make it hard on us. That doesn't mean that as women, you have to make things complicated while trying to get your needs met by men.

We are trying to be the team player you claim to have been looking for, when all the while you're allowing influences within your circle to dictate how you're going to incorporate men into your world. So I am here to say that you will never have a man come at you with the right approach of making things easier for you until you lose the attitude. Your tone and temperament is what got his attention in the first place. Quit letting society and your girlfriends tell you that a little attitude won't hurt anybody because it is hurting you and your chances with Mr. Right. Show them that you know what you're doing by letting him in on your true desire to let him make things easier for you. And that you will be right there to show him how much you really appreciate it. Because contrary to beliefs…

"We as men don't want to have to go through a STORM to get to a RAINBOW"

CHAPTER 4

"Prepping the Meal Before the Relationship"

There is nothing more satisfying than a meal that is well prepared. My mom was a master at preparing a good meal. She knew just the right ingredients and the perfect amount of "everything" to put into a meal. She also knew just the right amount of **"LOVE"**! I felt as though I was watching Mozart every time I watched her cook a meal and every time I watched her interact with my father. He was definitely a sucker for a good meal—which meant she had him at "hello" in more ways than one. As the years went by, I noticed a lot of things about my mom and dad's relationship, which has inspired many concepts in the book that you are currently reading. However, the one thing that always stood out to me was how present my dad was at meeting all my mom's needs and he never turned down a meal.

In reflection, I don't believe that I ever heard him even complain about a single meal. With that being said, my mom must have been one hell of a cook! It wasn't until I started asking my mom to teach me how to cook did I realize that it was not the cooking part that made the meal. It was the *prepping* that made the meal edible and good. It was the care and the attention to detail my mom brought to every meal that insured the meal was going to make its point with me, my dad and my two sisters. And I have to say, that she made that point consistently.

But these meals didn't come without me being curious because I noticed that she never used any cups to measure the ingredients of what she was making. So one day I asked her why she didn't use anything to measure the food. She told me that it was just like getting a man—and that as long as she was doing it with confidence and a desire to get it right the first time, it would never go wrong. And sure enough every meal turned out just fine for almost 38 years of my life. But it wasn't the 38 years in my life that was as important as her 26 years in my dad's life because she had showed me more about relationships cooking for him all those years than any relationship I have been in.

When I got older, my mom began to tell me about some of the things I had seen as a child between her and my dad. And one of those things that were evident to me was that my mom never learned how to drive, which I was puzzled about. I mean… There wasn't a person I knew who didn't know how to drive, with the exception of my mother! But when you have a true purpose and a good reason behind something, it almost makes you wonder why nobody else thought this way. But nobody did, except my mother, the master chef!

And I know! You ask…. What was so fascinating about his mother not learning how to drive? Well! It's not the being able to drive or not being able to drive that should bring on this question, but rather the fascinating reason behind it! So here goes. So many times when we start getting to know someone as we're dating, we have this tendency to think that letting things take a so-called natural course is the way to do things. But the question I would like to ask to you the reader is—what is the natural course when getting to know someone? Well! I have my own perspective on it, but I'm going to honor my mom by using hers, because honestly, it's a better perspective.

One day while talking to my mom about women she told me that if I was going to be successful with a woman, I was going to have to allow a woman to better prepare me for the desires and situations in her life. She also said that I would have to be open to being like a meal that was unseasoned and unprepared. Interestingly, when my mother shared this with me, I didn't really understand what she meant by this. Therefore, I asked her to please elaborate… and she did! She began to share with me stories of how my dad became excellent at meeting her needs. But it wasn't his meeting her needs that became the most fascinating part of the stories she shared with me. No, instead it was the way in which she prepared him to meet her needs that resonated with me from that moment until now. And even though it took me a while to understand why it was so important for me to allow a woman to come at me this way, my mom's words still resonate with me till this day.

So many times when talking to my sisters and some of the other females in my life, my mom would present them with the concept of preparing a man to be successful. She would give them little things to go on and look for—which would give them the indication whether this man would be edible if seasoned right, or did he have an expiration date and could not be used for future prepping. As the old saying goes, ".... you live and you learn," right? Well.... if it was that easy there would be no reason for me and all the other authors of inspiration to bring these concepts to the table. But it isn't! It is definitely something to be said about having the knowledge to make something complete. To make something good and to ultimately be impressed with the results! But what has been lost in translation is the process that has helped you get to that point. That is what is missing with most women of today.

You are missing the importance of preparing a man for the rigors that it is going to take to deal with you. You are missing the importance in preparing a man for the long haul you claim to want in a relationship. You are missing the importance in preparing a man to enjoy being successful at meeting your needs with flying colors. You are missing the importance of preparing a man so that your family and friends don't have an issue about him and/or your situation. You are missing the importance of preparing a man so that when you get to where things have become about routine, you're not missing out on your true desires in that routine. You are missing the importance of preparing a man so that he is confident in his ability to get it done. You are missing the importance of preparing a man so you don't have to keep telling him over and over again what to do.

When I began writing this book, one of the things that I found extremely disheartening was how unwilling most women were about making sure they got their needs met the way they saw fit. It's like an owner of a business hiring workers, not prepping them for the job at hand and then letting them do things their way and thinking they were going to get the job done. You and I both know that particular business would never last. I would even go one step further and say that there is nothing more disheartening than taking the advice from the females in your life—who has that same unwillingness to teach a man how to be successful. "But why should I have to prep him?" you women keep asking me and all the other people who have a problem with your lack of willingness. "Why should I have to prep him on knowing what I need instead of him just automatically knowing what I need?"

Well! Before I start answering your questions let me ask a few of my own. What is the point of getting to know a woman if she's already saying that we as men should already know how to meet her needs? I mean…. if that's the case, then why aren't we as men and women just bypassing the getting to know process and going right into a relationship? And why are we as men getting rewarded for using educated guesses when we're getting to know you and are ultimately being ridiculed in the relationship for those same educated guesses? I mean, if it was good enough for you to accept us that way when we were getting to know you, then why isn't it good enough for you when we get in a relationship with you? One of the things that I have learned about women when it pertains to desire is either a) you're benefiting from desire or b) you're complaining about it.

"But there would be no reason to complain about your desires if you were being responsible for how you got them met."

Because you and I both know that you would be complaining about **YOURSELF!** And being real with yourself is not the way you're doing things these days while you're trying to get us to be just as real. Being honest with yourself is not something that you're even used to doing because if you were, you would not have a problem getting your needs and desires met in the first place. Now to answer your questions from earlier about why women should have to teach a man or prep a man for a life with you is because not only does a man not know how you want things done, he knows that if he doesn't build some kind of foundation with you for the long haul, the bottom is going to eventually fall out. Most of you women are asking a man to build a foundation on his own and you're still not satisfied with the results. But he knew that in order for him to get the job for the long haul he was going to have to count on you to help him build that foundation.

Here it is, most of you women are leaving it up to a man to build a foundation, and then you resent the fact that what he has created is not sturdy enough. You didn't care about your position to prep him—so the floor could be built to your liking. And yet, you insist on expressing your frustration with the way the foundation turned out. And now, he's just as frustrated as you. And the only reason that he hasn't just given up on you and just said "screw it" is because he feels that he's at least going to get compensated for the work he put in before he is done with the roller coaster ride you have taken him on!

Now you're mad because not only does he not want to start over building another foundation for you or with you, but he is still coming over and having sex with you to make up for the work he put in trying to make the point that he was capable of making all the difference to a woman who wanted no part in the building process but only wanted to complain about it. And instead of telling him that you are and were wrong for not taking some kind of initiative and responsibility for how the foundation was built—you present him with an attitude after the fact because he is not giving you a "do over."

You wonder why he is still coming around because his demeanor and desire to do things your way now is not something that he is up for anymore. And you know this! But what you don't know is that his mind has told him that you could never compensate him enough for the beating he just took trying to be successful with you, and he is going to keep having sex with you and using up your resources until he sees fit, or until you get tired. You finally see his point and move on to the next guy—doing the same thing that stopped the guy you just got rid of from being successful. Your mind is telling you that you didn't like the other guy's way of doing things anyway—though you could have made all of the difference in the world by preparing him to be successful from the onset. And you wonder why you and the guy never got to a point where the meal (i.e., the relationship) ever got cooking!

And now you have returned to your old ways in the form of denial, ruining another potential mate—all the while burning up the kitchen *again*. The smoke is not even clear before you start cooking again with the next guy, who has no idea that your "cooking skills" are suspect. And even though his expiration date is not up on his ability to learn from being set in his ways, he doesn't realize that you are going to leave him out on the counter too long in the defrosting process because you haven't gotten over the first meal you just ruined. But you got to him just in time because he's better than the meal you just ruined. He had a longer expiration date; therefore, waiting for you to give him a chance is not an issue.

So now he is ready for you to prep him on how things are going to be at the start and hopefully for the duration of the time that he is going to be with you. But you take it upon yourself to call in a back-up chef called your "girlfriend" to put the seasoning on this guy because you already ruined one meal. And ruining two meals in this short of a time is not going to go over well with your psyche. Your girlfriend is excited because she has some "new seasonings" that she hasn't been able to use because she stopped buying groceries a long time ago and is out of touch on what to look for in men. You're a little apprehensive because you have never taken her advice before on how to deal with the male species. But ruining another potential mate with your prep skills will once and for all make the case that you are just a bad cook.

You keep telling yourself that this will work and that allowing your girlfriend to "prep" the meal that is your future mate—is going to yield results that are good and edible. However, there's only one problem: you never asked her what seasonings or approach she was going to use to insure that the meal was going to be edible and good this time. Never once did it cross your mind that you have not agreed to anything when it came to your taste in men. Until now, you've never even shared recipes. And now you're going to let her season a whole meal for you? She finally presents you with the ingredients, and you notice that everything on her list doesn't set well with you. But you go along with it anyway because nothing could be worse than the meal you just burned. Nothing could be worse than the man you just got rid of because you can't be that bad. He had already reached the expiration date when you took a chance on him.

And with that being said, while this man marinates on the ingredients that your friend passed down to you, you notice that you've become a little uncomfortable with the time that it has taken for him to understand how you want and need things done. But you were the one that thought that it was a good idea allowing your friend to prepare this man. And now, he isn't turning out right because you forgot that you are using your girlfriend's measuring cups and tools to insure that the meal comes out her way and not yours. You are using your girlfriend's beliefs and thoughts about her approach to men and now it is taking longer for him to understand you because it doesn't seem to fit you. You try to save your opinions and complaints for the finished product but you're not liking the smell of it. And now you notice that he is not getting done by the time your girlfriend said that he would be—according to her instruction of things.

You can't understand why he is not edible and ready to be in a relationship because you followed her ingredients to a tee. So you look over the ingredients again, all the while calling your girlfriend to make sure you followed her instructions correctly. But what you forgot to take into account is that your girlfriend has ruined many a meal with those same ingredients. That's why she was in NO position to pass them on to you! And now you ask yourself, "Why would my girlfriend give me some advice that's going to ruin another potential meal when she just saw me ruin one?" It's because she thinks that maybe you will do better than she did with that recipe. That a way! She can make the case with herself that she wasn't that bad of a cook after all, while helping you to find your culinary skills.

Never once did it cross her mind or your other girlfriend's minds who had been unsuccessful with that same recipe—that the meal was never going to turn out right using those ingredients and/or instructions together. And what keeps resonating with every failed attempt at prepping these men is that *you* have made everyone else responsible for how your meal turns out. So tell me, why aren't you taking the responsibility for prepping a man before the relationship? And why are you constantly blaming everyone else for how it turns out? There is an old saying that….

"You don't take chicken breast out of the freezer and just throw it in the oven. You have to prep it first (defrosting, seasoning, etc.,) so that the end result yields something edible *and* delicious."

A man is no different. You can't take us from a cold freezer and throw us into the fire of your lives and expect us not be tough pickings! You can't take us from one extreme to the next and expect us to be successful with you. Here it is! Most of you women are telling us that we have to take our time getting to know you. However, you're not doing your part in prepping us to insure that by the time we're done cooking we have something edible and good to go on. You have not followed your own instructions to give us the best chance to make our case, as I stated in the second chapter. But I will give you the benefit of the doubt and say that perhaps the instructions you are going on are not good for your way of doing things. Or perhaps you just need to accept the fact that you are going to burn every meal you cook and let those women who have culinary skills benefit from your generosity. Either way, most of you need to go back to the drawing board, (culinary school) reinventing yourselves and your ideals or put your knives away forever!

Now just because you're not good at prepping a man doesn't mean that you are no good at training one. Maybe you are in the wrong field and you just needed to find your niche. The problem with most people is we are so stuck on one way of doing things that we don't bother to truly acknowledge what we are good at. Maybe your thing is not prepping a man, but training one. Maybe your thing is being able to say what needs to be done and have it be done as such instead of having to actually show a man by example how to do it. That doesn't mean that he is going to be any less prepared with your way of doing things. I know that teaching a man what your needs are has, on occasion, been a tiresome quest because most women feel like a man should already know how to treat a woman. But what I will say to that is….

"ALL DOGS DON'T GO TO HEAVEN, SO YOU BETTER TRAIN'EM"

When someone is taking on any assignment in life, the first thing that is provided to guarantee the person's success is an "example" or "training." This could be anything from on the job training, to an example of how something works that we have purchased in a store or even handy work that is performed around the house. We are always provided with an example and training so that things can unfold according to plan. In the getting to know process—at times we have a tendency to take a person from A to C, skipping the "B" part, where the training or examples were! So many times I have seen relationships fail because neither one of the participants received the proper training that would have made the transition from getting to know each other into the relationship a much easier process. Every woman has the opportunity to prepare a man for a life with her. But not only do you not train him for your desires, but then you complain when he is not passing your test with flying colors.

A fireman does not train for one day and then is thrown into a forest fire. Some of you women are throwing these men into the forest fire of your lives with no survival training. Aside from this, he's not even your man yet and has no business being caught up in the cross fire! One of the things that made my mom and dad's relationship go according to her plan, was my mom took the time to train and prepare my dad for the ultimate success in consistently meeting her needs—and I would highly recommend that you do the same. Not only should you be ready to train the man you are dating, and provide consistent examples of how you want and need things done, but you should be grading him on his ability to do so.

Some of you reading this book may protest, simply stating, "But I like him, Tonee!" But I know that you like him. That does not mean that you don't put him to the test before you decide to give him a higher position in your life. And it definitely doesn't mean that as women, you should be given a pass on how you grade his work ethic and the things that you claim is going to make the decision for you. So how many of you are taking the time to prep or train a man to be successful in your lives? How many of you are even taking responsibility for it?

Interestingly, when I have brought this point to a forum of women, there was one comment that got my attention more than all others. One young woman asked me if I knew what she should be asking men to do at the start in order for her to make a conscious decision on making him her man. I told her that it was not my job or any other man's job to tell her what she needed out of a man. That she should know more than me or any other man what she needed in order to be okay with giving that man his position in her life. That's when the light bulb went off in my head. It was right at that moment in the middle of this forum that I realized that most women not only don't know what they need out of a man, but don't know what they are grading him on based on that not knowing. Not only are you not prepping a man to be the person you need him to be, but you are not grading him correctly based on the things that you claim to want out of him. So my question to you is….

"How are you grading the men you're letting into your life?"

How are you grading the potential of a man when everything you've been taught by this New Age way of thinking has encouraged women to disregard this process entirely? I don't understand how you can be a woman who says that "actions speak louder than words" and not have the ability to grade a man on what he does as opposed to what he says.

When I look at my sisters, one of the things that I noticed about them in their younger years when dealing with men, was how bad they were at not only picking a man, but grading him on his performance when it came to meeting their needs. It was a concept that was being continuously looked over and not seen as the sole reason why their perceptions about men would later be tainted. And they are not alone! Most women have created a negative perception about men because they have not graded him correctly on his ability and desire to meet their needs. And furthermore, they have not gotten rid of him in a timely manner to insure that their perceptions about men would not be tainted.

On numerous occasions, I have seen the women in my life or women in other situations being with a man that was incapable of doing nothing or not being with the man that was capable of doing everything. But there was one woman who knew better. My mom! She knew that she had to get rid of a man in a timely fashion to insure that she was not going to take negativities into the next encounter she had with the next man. Even when she would tell the other women in my life why they needed to get rid of a man in a timely fashion, they would still keep these men around.

I mean, Stevie Wonder could see that there was nothing about these men that said these women should have been taking a chance on them, but they did. Even as I write this, there are many of you out there right now who are taking a chance on a man that you have not graded with high marks, however, you continue to allow him to be in your life. Many of you are taking chances on a man you have not graded correctly because you don't know what you are supposed to be grading him on.

Why are you having sex with this man? Why are you hanging out with this person as long as you have? You are on the verge of being pregnant by a man who has shown you nothing but some strokes on your way to parenthood. "But I am giving him a chance to get his act together, Tonee?" I understand that you're giving him a chance to prove himself but he has had plenty of time for you to realize that he was a

"crash dummy" waiting to happen. In the meantime, you have a good guy waiting in the wings to pick up where he left off, but you keep telling yourself that he will come around because you're better off with him than without him. You have even sold yourself on the thinking that if nothing else, you can always play victim if it doesn't work out.

But the jury is out on you already! And even though society will give you the victim's role, I am here to say that I am doing no such thing. As a matter of fact, I am doing the opposite by telling you that it is definitely all your fault that you haven't taken his potential at face value. I would even go out on a limb and ask you if you even know what you are looking for in a man when you are grading him on his potentials? You call yourself a woman who has the ability to get a man to do what you want. And yet! You have gone along with his lack of desire and willingness to do what is required of him.

At the end of the day, a man is in no position to dictate to you how he is going to do things. Right! He will never be able to play games on you because you have made it all about *your* way of doing things, especially at this time in the process where he is getting to know you! Right! You are the one who is in the driver's seat! But ever since he got in your life he has been using you as the crash dummy, and your excuse for this is that he talked a good game. He made everything sound good at the start. But you're a woman who says that....

"Actions speak louder than words."

And yet you feed us the excuse that he made everything sound good. But in the same breath, you said that you didn't go on words more than actions. So why all of a sudden now that I challenge what you said, you feed me a concept that you claimed that you aren't going on? Why the sudden change? Are you giving me an excuse or are you one of those women who goes on what you've heard other women say? You have no clue as to what you're talking about, do you? Here you are letting this man force feed you the words you claim not to be going on and then blame him for the fact that you're not doing your homework on him. Don't be mad at me that I took away the victim's role from you and replaced it with you finally seeing that he didn't play a game on you more than you played the game on yourself. Don't be mad at me that you don't get to hide from the responsibility that you have been awarded when dealing with men from the start.

Shame on you! You knew that he was incapable, but you took a chance on him anyway. You definitely would have taken credit if he was "the one" and the relationship would have worked out. So why aren't you taking the blame for the fact that he was a nobody from the start? At least not for you! You don't get it both ways. You don't get to take credit for things when they work out and then play victim when they don't. But I don't want to totally make it sound like all women are like this. But for the most part, I have seen time and time again where the women who take chances on these kinds of men want society to overlook the fact that her ability to pick a man is suspect. And I have to say that….

"It seems to be more about "survival" than "common sense" that some of you have taken chance after chance on men who had no business being in your lives."

So needless to say that my mom knew what her business was when it came to my dad. She knew that the meal was never going to turn out to be edible and good unless she put the time in preparing and training my dad to be there the way she desired him to be. And nothing could have made this point more than my mom not learning how to drive because 1) it fed my dad's ego to know that she needed him that way; 2) She knew where he was at all times, so there was no way that he could be doing it somebody else's way. Well, leave it up to my mom to always have a recipe for success.

CHAPTER 5

"Help me… Help you!"

Oftentimes, I hear women talk about wanting a relationship that's 50/50, but I have come to realize that's simply not the case. As a matter of fact, from the moment you meet a man up until the day you get married, the man is usually fitting the bill. But what if a man told you that……

"He was tired of taking care of you. That he wants to be taken care of for a change?"

What would your answer be? Since the days of Adam and Eve, God created Eve to be a help mate for Adam. However, looking at the way things are today, it seems that God's desire for a woman to be a help mate to a man has fallen on very deaf ears. Usually when I bring up this question of helping to a forum of men and women, it gets mixed reviews in the area of how that help is provided. There are various ways in which men and women help and support one another. But the one that always seem to make things uncomfortable with men and women is the financial aspect of help. This has always been the touchiest subject to bring up, asking a woman to help a man in order for them to help her.

When you think about it, it's like a slap in the face that men who have been taking care of women since the dawn of time is having a hard time getting women to reciprocate the love. I mean… just on that fact alone—one would think that a woman would be happy to reciprocate the love. Just by that fact alone-one would think that a woman would have no problem going out of her way for a man that has shown her that he deserves it. But women are saying "Not so fast…I'm not giving him anything. As a matter of fact, if he's not coming with the same amount as me, or more, I'm not even dealing with him." There is an old saying that "Money can't buy you love." But when it comes to a woman in this era—it can sure buy you some time. Time to get your act together the way women see fit. Isn't that right, ladies?

Honestly, women should be the first to understand when a man doesn't want to pay for dinner because you're capable of buying your own dinner. You should understand when a man wants to pressure you into having sex because he has spent quite a bit of his hard earned money on you. You should understand when you may have to pay for drinks because his card is maxed out from wining and dining you all week. I mean… why should you be able to just show up and not have to do anything to let him know that you are going to be there for him when times get rough?

It amazes me how the man is the one taking all the risk while you benefit from his so called independence and your own. Where is the trade-off? It's not like you're going to sleep with him on the first date to show that you appreciate it, if at all. So why does a man have to sacrifice for a woman who is playing it safe with him? That same woman that came at you with the "I believe a relationship is 50/50" is watching you wine and dine her like it's the Last Supper and not so much as a piece of lint has fallen out of her purse or pocket to let you know that she will be willing to help when the situation presents itself.

In all honesty, I have been called a "player" by quite a few women because I have demanded out of women the same things that they have demanded out of me. Men are putting themselves out there just as much as women—in good faith that their effort and resources won't be taken for granted. He must feel as though he's not being taken for a ride too. Just like you want to know that if you give of yourself, he's not going to disrespect you and take you for granted.

So why is society still putting man in an old school tradition of being the provider when women are approaching men with this new school mentality that a man doesn't have to be in that role?

I hear women all of the time boasting that they can take care of themselves and that they don't need a man to take care of them. But yet, they take advantage of an old school tradition that by my observation needs to be revised to today's way of approaching the getting to know process. Please help me to understand why men still have to carry a burden set by tradition, when women are not fulfilling their position as set by the same tradition? Given the economic climate of our country, the ignorance displayed by some women to think that every man should be successful is a bit unrealistic. Women are holding men in general to a standard that cannot be achieved by every single man—especially if he's got to do it on his own, which God never intended.

They are a lot of men out here who could help a woman, if a woman took the time to help him. The sole reason for your existence is based on this point because God knew that man was not going to be able to do it alone. God knew that the extra motivation a woman brings to a man was going to be very vital to his makeup. And if you women out there in society took the time to sacrifice for a man in the way that he is willing to sacrifice for you, the relationship would automatically take on a natural course of success. These opinions and findings are not only subjected to my way of thinking because I have seen so many of my friends go through this observation in their situations with women where they were the only ones taking all the risk while the women were playing it safe. "But he's the man, Tonee! He should be doing those things."

"Why should he take all of the risk simply because he's the man?"

Why should he be taking all the risk while women get to play it safe? And why do you as women feel that you don't have to take any risks?

Where is the trade off here? Where in a man's dealings with you are you going to show him that you are taking risk beyond him just being in your presence? Oftentimes, my sisters will ask me about men and why so many men are selfish in their approach with women. Well! If you women really look at it from a logical stand point, a lot of the behavior that man is displaying these days has to do with the way that some women operate in their selfishness towards men. They have learned from the best.

With that being said, I know that some women are going to come with the most extreme of circumstances to prove the point of why they are playing it safe with a man who is sacrificing everything to be with you. It has always been the tactic of choice with some women who are in denial to come up with the most extreme of circumstances to validate their reasons or what I call **"excuses."** A man has got to know that you are in his corner! And it doesn't put him at ease that every time he has asked you for something that there is a pause for concern. I have witnessed so many cases where a woman have had the opportunity to help a man, help them. But they felt that not only was it not worth it, but they would play on his manhood to make their point. There is old saying that…

"Behind every good man there is a good woman"

I will take it even further and say that behind every good man there is a woman helping him to become that way. She is not sitting in the wings until he figures it out on his own. It's easy for us as human beings not to see the potential in something or someone, especially if it means that we have to make a sacrifice for it. Oftentimes, it's not in our nature to make sacrifices for family, much less a stranger. But men we have to get better! We have to get better at telling these women that we need their help in order to be the men they want us to be. And women need to start seeing that we can't be the men you need us to be without that help.

"Identify the small minded people in your life and get rid of them."

Don't deal with them. Use your energy proving to them that they made a mistake on you. Find a woman who wants to be the reason why you have made it this far. Find a woman who sees your potential and is not afraid to tap into it for her own benefit! You are more than what those other women say about you. So concentrate on the woman who is making the effort to help you so you can help her. Most women can't see your potential because they are going on everything else but your heart! It's always fascinating to me to hear women talking about having a man with a good character, and yet you're not helping him to tap into that part of himself. You're not helping him to see that you are going to be just as much of an intricate part of his life and makeup as he is going to be of yours. You're not helping him to see that you're going to show him that you're not in it just for your own gain—but his as well. That it is not just a "me" thing more than it is a "we" thing.

One of the things that resonated with me as a child growing up was how willing my mom was to put herself in harm's way to prove to my dad that she was in it for the long haul. She was the one who took it upon herself to put my dad in a frame of mind that was going to have him thinking how he ever took a chance on any other woman in his life. That's the kind of woman you should be aspiring to be because that's the kind of woman every man is looking for. The kind of woman who makes us feel like it is "you and me against the world." The kind of woman that makes us feel like it is you and me against all odds.

Most of the successful relationships I have witnessed over the years are because of a woman who declared that she was going to help her man achieve the level that is going to benefit, not only his moving forward, but their moving forward together. I knew women who had this kind of attitude throughout my younger years. But as I have grown older, I have seen this kind of woman dwindle. I have even seen the concept itself dwindle. As men we feel that women are no longer using their energy to help us become better men for them. And they wonder why we are no good at it. You wonder why the men that you are taking chances on are no good at helping you with your desires when you're not helping motivate his ability to do so.

The days of women staying home and raising the kids seems to be all but a distant memory in our society today. Today, we are told that we need a two income household if we're ever going to keep up with the Jones's. Therefore, most kids are not being raised with the upbringing that I was raised with back when my mom stayed home and carried out her position as a help mate to my dad. It's also fair to say that women have changed their perception and interpretation with the whole independent woman approach, making me and all the rest of mankind think that this was something that was going to help us in the long run. But if we look at it for what it really is…. it has done nothing but bring out the aggressiveness in women because we have brought on more of a competitive nature when getting to know each other. There is no more team concept. There is no more "cheerleader to jock" mentality anymore. And this is what we are selling to the next generation of women?

We are selling the next generation of young ladies on the fact that they don't have to help a man to become a better man when they can use that energy to help themselves to become a better woman. But what is not being told to these young ladies is that a man will be resentful in his quest to be the man you want him to be. And if you're not up for helping a man to become better at meeting your requirements, then expect him to be less of one for you. As a man, you need to get women to understand that you are not taking their position lightly and that you want the same respect in return.

"Get them to understand that you are more than what they settle for in themselves…"

Get women to understand that if they are not going to help you then why should they benefit. Get them to understand that if they are not going to help you, then they should not be included in anything that you have going on in your life. Get them to understand that you don't have time for a woman who has no desire to use her resources to help you to become what she has always wanted in a man. Otherwise, do what men do and move on to the next woman who you feel is ready and willing to help you, help her.

Now as statistics shows, there are a lot of young men and women being raised in single parent homes these days. This means that a majority of these children are being raised by their mother, who plays the most important part of their development. She is the one that interpret for her sons and daughters the rules and regulations they are going to live by and usually go by once they become adults themselves. She is the one that will normally give her sons and daughters their so called makeup. It's not often that she will ask or even allow most men to play any type of role in the development of her children. Especially, if she's getting to know them! And yet, the minute that child doesn't succeed who is the person that usually gets blamed most of the time for how that child has ended up? It's the person who had the least amount of interaction with them—and normally that's a man.

As a young man, I found myself at times struggling with my identity as a man because I had bought into the cliché that my odds of being successful were going to be less than my chances of being successful because my father was not there to teach me. But I had it all wrong because my mother helped a man, help her to raise me. There are a lot of women that are not helping a man, help them to teach these children how to act in society, let alone respect people. And we wonder why so many children have emotional and developmental issues. We wonder why so many children can't handle having to be accountable for anything. I was one of those children at one time who were having a hard time when my mother was single because she was not allowing a man to help her with me. She was not allowing a man to show me what being responsible for something was all about. And so, I took in all the negative stereotypes that came with being in a single parent home. I took in all the anger, the resentments, the frustrations and most of all…. the abandonment of not having a male around because my mother was not allowing men to help her, with me.

Then something changed! My mom had stopped blaming men for her place in life and started taking some responsibility for the fact that she was bringing a single-minded approach for the longest time with men. I could see that she was tired of doing it all by herself. I could sense that she was tired of being alone. I could tell that she was ready to help a man, help her with raising me and my two siblings. And even though at times, my stepfather wasn't the best teacher that I could have hoped for, there was a man there for me to at least get a glimpse of how things were supposed to be with me and my future mate. I was learning…. But what about you!

There are so many women that are making it seem like to your children that it is okay being alone. There are so many women that are making it seem like to your children that it is okay trying to raise a household by yourself. There are so many women that are making it seem like it is a man's fault that you are not showing them what it looks like to be in a relationship with someone. There are so many women that are making it seem like your children's relationship aren't going to suffer because they have never seen a man loving you the right way. Your children haven't even seen you with another man after your divorce.

And yet! You claim to love your children and their well-being. But nothing about the way you are approaching life or a man is showing them that you know what you're doing. That's why they want you to get back with their father because an abusive man is better than no man at all. And now! Your children are getting older and you realize that they're going to be going to college soon and you will be in the house all by yourself hearing yourself echo. You've been out of the dating game for a while now because you took a few years off from dating to concentrate on raising them. You needed them for clarity. But now it's not so clear anymore why you took so much time to allow a man into your life and theirs. It's not so clear anymore why you allowed yourself to be so complacent about your desire for a man. But now you have a new found energy for something new.

So you buy into internet dating because even though you have a moment here and there, you don't have a lot of time to spend trying to get to know all types of men. But what other option is there? Right!

So you make plans to let your children in on your desire to find a man. You think your children are going to be happy for you but they're not because they think that your time spent looking for a man is going to interfere with the fact that they have had you at their beck and call for the past 5 years. So why the sudden change? They don't understand that for the last 5 years you have fought through loneliness at times. They don't understand that for the last 5 years you have second guessed yourself about divorcing their father because you miss the closeness. They don't understand that for the last 5 years you have felt more like a mother more than a woman who is in her sexual prime and you need a man to show you a good time. You couldn't be more excited about the possibility of finding someone to fulfill the 5 year hole in your heart. But you've been out of the dating game for a while now. And the women in your age group are not acting like they necessarily need men anymore. The women in your age group and in other age groups are not helping men, help them.

As men we have been taught all of our lives to be a team player and show a woman that we are ready to help women be the women that they have aspired to be. Not letting a man help you, so you can help him is not going make things harder for men. It's going to make things harder on you as women. It's going to make things even harder on your children. They are the ones that are not benefiting from the team player concept because you are raising them in a single-minded environment. It's something that I learned from my mom and dad at any early age, to be a team player and understand the concept of thinking and caring about somebody other than myself. It didn't dawn on me until I got older how important that team concept was going to be in every part of my life. As women, you don't understand that not helping a man, help you to teach your children what being a team player is all about is setting them up to have certain issues that wouldn't necessarily be there if they weren't being raised in a single-minded environment.

When I look at the world today, I see more children that are more selfish than ever. I see more children that are unprepared to deal with situations that have a team concept in them because they were raised in a single-minded environment. As parents, we are the ones that our children are going to get their development from. Their examples from! Their substance from! You women that are raising your children in a single-minded environment don't understand the disservice you're doing to your children for giving them the indication that you're okay not letting a man help you, help them. You women don't realize that you are doing your children a disservice not letting them see what "LOVE" is really like between you and a man. Your children long for it more than you will ever know. Your children long for seeing you happy with someone that can lay down the examples and values they are going to live by in their lives. Your children long for that attention that comes with knowing that someone beyond mom cares about them. Your children long for how all the children in the neighborhood will love coming to your house because the other children can't wait to see this man that everybody has been talking about that's in your life and theirs. It means that much to them.

But all the while, you have listen to society and the people around you tell you that it's not appropriate letting your children see men coming in and out of your house and bed. And as well you shouldn't. But when are you going to jumpstart your heart again to show a man that you not only care about your desires but your children's desires as well by having him around? When are you going to jumpstart your heart to show a man that you want to show your children what being a team player is all about? All this time, you thought that "LOVE" was eluding you. But it was you that was eluding "LOVE". It was you who took the stance that you could be just as okay without it more than you are with it. It was you who took the stance that you were going to allow the lack of desire in others interfere with your desire to want something special.

Every year that has gone by up until now, you don't realize has put your children in a no win situation. Every year that has gone by up until now has put your children behind in learning what true "LOVE" is like. Every year that has gone by has put your children in a single-minded way of thinking because you have not given them that everyday example in your life. And now that you have used the "independent" woman concept to justify your being alone, they are even more confused than they were when you were in your unhealthy relationship with their father.

They see you as this great mom and nothing else because you have stopped them from seeing all the other special qualities in you. They haven't seen you as a team player in a long time. They have never seen you as a lover because you didn't marry their dad for that more than the financial aspect of living. That's why it's so easy for you to jump on all the other single-minded women's bandwagon when it comes to the "independent" woman concept. They have never seen you in support of a man. They have never seen you motivate, encourage or inspire one. And so! This is how you're going to send them out into the world? Uninformed and unprepared to fulfill some man or woman's life with "LOVE" and a willingness to be a team player! You couldn't do them a worse disservice than not helping a man, help you show your children the examples that only "LOVE" could show.

These young men out in society! They don't have a clue as to what their responsibility is supposed to be with a young lady because you never brought a man around them so they could see first hand the bond between you. Most of you don't even share your good experiences with men to your sons, so that when he leaves your household he has some kind of clue as to how he should be approaching the opposite sex. Instead, you believe that shielding your son and/or sons from your relationship with a man and not allowing him and/or them to see you with a man is going to be better for their make ups in the long run. Did it ever occur to you that not letting them see a man taking on that responsibility for you and them is going to give them the false sense that they can go out and get a girl pregnant and if it doesn't work between them—they feel that the child will be just fine being raised by the mom alone because you raised them the same way? Did it ever occur to you that not allowing your daughter and/or daughters seeing you with a man is going to give them a false sense that they don't need one? I mean… you claim to love your children.

But nothing you have shown them about finding a good man or being with one has been a part of their upbringing. Nothing about finding a good man or being with one has been a part of your conversations with them. They don't know the energy and stress that it takes to be both the mommy and daddy for them. They don't understand the loneliness that will present itself to them if they go about the finding a mate this way. God blessed you with those children because he knew that you had it in you to teach them. God blessed you with those children because he knew that you had it in you to be a role model and good example for them. God blessed you with those children because he knew that you had it within your heart to show them what being in "LOVE" was all about.

But you have not used yourself as the motivating factor for a man in a long time. You have not used yourself as a commodity in a long time. You have not used yourself as the prize in a long time. You can't even remember the last time you were excited about a man. But now the moment of truth is here for you to put yourself back out in the dating scene. You have so many emotions going through you as you create a profile on a couple of dating sites to see if there are some potential mates and/or possibilities! But after being on there for little over a month, you realize the energy and effort that it takes just to weed out the people you're not attracted to or anything in common with, let alone find the next "LOVE" of your life. Not to mention, subjecting your children to another failed relationship.

So you start to listen to the little voice in your head ask you "is this really worth it?" Is this whole thing really worth getting your hopes up and your children's hopes up, only to be disappointed by a man again? I mean, you know that you can handle it. But what about your children? What are they going to think if you allow a man to come and ruin the stability you and them have created over the last 5 years? What are they going to think if this man ends up being worse than their dad, only fueling their thoughts and desires that you should have stayed with him?

All these things have gone through your mind as you scroll through profile after profile on the dating site, disappointed by the men you have come across. That is when Mr. "Oh My God" crosses your screen. You don't know where he came from but you're happy because you haven't felt this alive in a long time. You send him a flirt then an email, hoping that he feels the same way about you. Your children don't know why you have this extra kick in your step today but they like it. They don't know that you are looking forward to getting back online to see if you got a response from Mr. "Oh My God". You're excited! And after a long day, you rush home to see if your prayers have been answered or your disappointments have been confirmed. But God was listening. Not only does Mr. "Oh My God" send you an email but he sends you an email that sounds like a man who wants you just as much as you want him.

You exchange a couple more emails to get comfortable with each other so you can make the next step of talking on the phone. Finally, the day has come for you to talk on the phone and you decide to meet each other for dinner so you can confirm your findings. The date goes on without a "hitch". He has shown you the time of your life. You walk into the house floating on air because you had a good night. But reality sets in when that little voice in your head tells you that you have to tell the kids about him. But before you do, you want to go on a couple more dates to confirm that he is not just a man looking for another notch to put on his belt. That he is not looking for another victim to entertain his friends at the gym with. He has made it through all your tests and you thought that you were ready to have him meet the children. You think that it is still too soon to be bringing your children into the mix but he is pushing the envelope because he wants you to know that he can handle it. That is when your single-minded way of doing things presents itself. That is when your single-minded way of doing things say that "why can't we get to know each other some more before he sees my children? I don't think that they are ready to meet another man yet because they haven't gotten over me not being with their father."

But as women, what you don't understand is your children have made your finding a man or not finding a man, about them more then you. They have made it about them because you have given them a right to speak on your desire's behalf. They don't know what's best for you or them. And now that you have a man that could help you, help them, you're getting cold feet. Once again, you would rather be what you consider to be comfortable in being wrong than uncomfortable in being right. You would rather allow your children to ruin the possibility of "LOVE" rather than accept the fact that you may have to choose his side and make things a little unstable for everyone involved. You have taken the easy way out the last 5 years. And now that you may have to do some work into changing the mindset of your household to include this man, it doesn't seem like it is a formidable reason to do so.

That is when you start to make up stories and excuses to sabotage moving forward with Mr. "Oh My Gosh". You have made him just as confused with your recent approach because you don't want to tell him that it is really because of your children that you are finding it hard to move forward with him. But he knows! And now he is seeing you in your childlike state while you allow your children to take on the role of parent. You don't understand why he is moving further and further away from you and your way of doing things. You think that the reasons that you have given him for slowing things down with him are justified. But you never took into account how bad you look to a man when you allow your children to dictate his future with you and your future with him.

So you tell me, when are you going to help a man, help you with your children and have them see that their opinions about your desire to be with a man is more about you than them? When are you going to help a man, help you with getting close to them? Not teaching a man and helping him to be involved with your children is only going to hurt you and them in the long run. One of the most ironic clichés is that some of these men have come from households like your sons and daughters who have been raised with their moms not letting them see her interact with a man as well. That is why he is pushing the envelope to get to know them.

"Even if you are a single parent, that doesn't mean that you have to be single-minded."

A lot of women have brought a single-minded approach to the table with men, and then are baffled that men take them for granted. However, as I previously stated, men are in no position to dictate to you when they haven't been given a position to do so yet. But they are in a position to mock or mimic what you do. That is why we have bought into that independent woman concept because we feel that there is no need to fight you on a concept you don't believe in, especially if it doesn't stop us from getting our needs met. But a real man who believes in the "help me, help you" concept knows that agreeing with that single-minded approach is going to have you ridiculing his position the same way you did the guy before him, and the guy before him! And so on and so forth.

That is why so many men agree with this single-minded approach is because they know that this is going to get them in a lot quicker than if they stayed in their true element and character to show you that they're going to be in it for the long haul. This single-minded approach has created a tunnel vision type mentality in you that has you and your children suffering the consequences from your ignorance. Once again, you have given your sons the indication that their baby's mother will be just fine raising little Jr. by herself. Once again, you have given your daughters the indication that they will be okay raising little Jr. on their own. But how could you know this single-minded approach was going to hurt you and your children? I mean….. no man has ever challenged you to see that being this way has done just that! But I am hear to say that if you're not going to help a man be the example your children have been looking for, then why should you be mad when he doesn't turn out that way? My mom used to always say that…

"When a person needs help the last thing they want is advice"

As men, we are no different. We are asking women for help! But instead of helping us help you, most women question our manhood in that request. Most women talk bad about a man the minute they feel that he can't do it all by himself. But what you don't understand is that God never intended for man to do it all by himself. Otherwise, what was the reason for creating you in the first place? Your whole existence is based in this fact that we cannot even make our point to God without having you there to validate it. So you better start understanding that….

"There is no way that we as men and women will ever be able to fully please God without helping each other with

the fact…. that we were never meant to do it ALONE"

That is why men ask for your help in everything that has to do with you because they are trying to create a child proof and fail proof solution so that they can be confident in their positions in your life. My mom built up my dad's confidence by helping him to find his way with us. By telling him about our dislikes and likes, our tendencies and quirks! She knew that he was going to be at his best as long as she helped a little bit along the way. If it's one thing that I can say that I pick up on right away about women is their willingness or unwillingness to help me be successful with them and everything that has to do with them from the start. And you men out there should be doing the same. You should always be asking a woman for her help in any and everything that you know is going to make getting to know her and being with her, easier. . But most of all, you should be requesting her help because you want her to feel like she's

INCLUDED!

So when are you going to start helping men teach your children that there is something wrong with being both the man and the woman in your own life? When are you going to start helping men, help you show the world that they made a mistake when they said that a man was not a necessity to a child's upbringing? When are you going to start helping men, help you show that with the right guidance—traditional relationships can and do exist? When are you going to start helping bridge the gap between men and women? When are you going to start helping men to create a **"LOVE"** that is unconditional so that you're sending emotional and mentally healthy children out into the world? When are you going to start helping men find the true joy in being with you? When are you going to start helping men, help you know that when it's all said and done you gave the best to one another—of what God gave to you? When are you going to start helping men, help you so that when you leave this earth, God is waiting to tell you "That was a job well done, my child!"

CHAPTER 6

Trial and Error

When we take a chance on something and it doesn't work out we usually move on to make it better the next time. Our family and friends don't usually question our judgment or our desire to see if it was going to work or not because they feel at least you gave it a try. Whether it was switching jobs to make better money, changing your hairdo to give yourself a new look, or maybe buying a new car that broke down on you, nobody would ridicule or complain about the fact that at least you took a chance to see if it was the best thing for you. This is what I refer to as **trial and error**. This is what enables me to keep situations that didn't turn out "right" in my life in a balanced perspective.

When I look at the world today, one of things that I find fascinating is how quickly we are to report the mistakes of one another, and are less inclined to report those decisions that did work out favorably. Failure has become the constant topic of the day whereas success is constantly being considered as back page news. With Google, Twitter and all the other media outlets available to ridicule and judge every mistake we make, we have created a society that has become very unsympathetic to trial and error. We have created a society that for whatever reason can't accept the fact that sometimes things don't go according to plan. Sometimes things just don't work out. Even when we have accepted this fact with most things in life, the one thing that we seem to go a different route on is the interaction between men and women. It wasn't until I began writing this book did I realize that most of the time….

"women are being ridiculed before they choose a man and men are being ridiculed after they choose you as their man".

A woman is being ridiculed before her decision whereas men are being ridiculed afterwards. It made me realize why some of my relationships and so many of yours are not working out. However, it wasn't the working out or not working out that brought on this curiosity that made me want to know why it was so hard for us as men and women to move on from something that didn't work to something that could and would. And so I decided to ask a couple of my male and female friends why they thought that it was so hard to move on to something successful with the next person after being unsuccessful with the person before.

It was enlightening to hear them all tell me that it was not difficult for them to move on from a man or woman, if only it affected them. Not understanding what they meant at the time I had to ask them to elaborate on this statement. And what I came to understand was that their family and friends were taking their situations and relationships more personal than they were. It made them feel as though they would never find someone that everybody would be satisfied with. They would never accept the trial and error part of you because they were taking it very personal that you keep failing at your attempts with "LOVE".

It's like a parent who raises a child who never got in trouble, but then the child leaves home and can't stay out of trouble. They take it personally because they think that their children's actions reflect their parenting skills. In essence, they think that their friends and family will label them as being "bad parents" rather than just having a child who has chosen to do things his or her own way as a grown up. The same thing goes with your failed attempts at finding "LOVE". Your friends and family take your failed attempts personally because they think that if you can't get it right then what chance do they have at getting it right, themselves. They look at your trial and error as failure and not as a bump in the road. They look at your trial and error as mistakes instead of taking into account that someone else has to play their role as well. They look at your trial and error as a continuous cycle that you will never break instead of a growing up process.

They don't understand you not being ready for something serious. They don't understand your desire to just have fun. You are in your late 30's, early 40's. How long does it take for you to grow up, because they need to know! They need to know if that's how long it's going to take them to find their true love or if your life is just an isolated incident to the way they feel they should be doing things. The only reason why your friends and family continue to give you a hard time about every man or woman you take a chance on is because they are looking for an answer to their issues about men and women themselves. You raised them to be good at relationships. And yet, you've been through two marriages before their high school graduation. You gave your friends advice on how they should act, talk and walk when interacting with men. And still, they have yet to see a good example of how it works for you.

You have told your girlfriends how they should never be vulnerable to a man. And yet, you have fallen madly in love with every man that has shown you a little bit of attention. You have become the opposite of what you say. You have not backed up your words with your actions. That is why they don't trust your judgment anymore. That is why they are no longer taking advice from you. Your family and friends are frustrated with you because you're not living up to the potentials they see in you for them to have a good example to live by. You knew that finding love and having love find you were going to take time. But you made it all sound simple. And now time is running out. It's not as easy to them as you made it seem. You have not put their minds and hearts at ease because you have not told them about the trial and error they were going to have desiring and finding love. You have not put their hearts and minds at ease by letting them know that it was okay to fail as long as their hearts were in the right place.

If it's one thing that we struggle with as men and women when it comes to relationships is accepting the fact that we are going to have trial and error in our lives more than we care to admit. If we don't start teaching and accepting the fact that we are going to have trial and error in our lives, we will never be able to move on with confidence and the belief that the next thing will work out. We will never be able to show the people in our lives a character that will help them in the long run. I go into every situation thinking that it is going to work. Now whether it turns out that way or not is another story. That doesn't mean that I have to acknowledge the failure of it any more or less than acknowledging the success of it. I don't even have to acknowledge the fact that the people in my life were proud of me when it worked and disappointed in me when it didn't. That's what people will do to you. They will be proud of you when things are making them look good and disappointed in you when they think the decision and/or decisions you have made are making them look bad. They will make it seem like your success was a result of their advice and support, while the failure was of your own doing.

One of the things that I am currently teaching my children is that I love them no matter what. That I will not be disappointed with the trial and error in their lives! I will never feel as though their mistakes and decision was based on anything I did or didn't do when raising them. Now, I'm not saying that I am supporting them in their wrong doing. However, I am saying that as a father, a friend, brother, neighbor, son and all the other positions I hold in my life, that I will always be a person who will be sympathetic to trial and error. And just for the record… if you hear someone saying that they don't want any drama in their life, don't deal with them because they will be the first person to ridicule and tear you down for the trial and error in your life.

The people in your life will even make a valiant effort to disregard the fact that the two of you were ever close, if at all. They will distance themselves as far as they can from the trial and error in your life. But not before they make sure that they have made the case with everyone around them that they were an unwilling participant in your game to ruin your life and theirs; and that it was a set up that they took absolutely no part in. In short, you have been carrying them this whole time and this is the thanks you get for at least trying to make something work when they haven't been in anything serious since the Pointer Sisters were on top of the charts!

All this time they have been riding your coat tails! And just when things start to get hectic, not only do they not give you a word of encouragement, but they then try to give you a word of advice. But the truth of the matter was they never had your back in the first place. They were just hanging around to play on your success or make themselves look good in your misery. Nothing has ever worked for them when it came to relationships and they can't handle the trial and error that comes with the territory. Yes! There are some people who think that they are entitled to something successful when nothing about their belief system brings on that fact. Nothing about the way they do things will ever bring on that kind of result. And this is who you have as a friend? This is who is mentoring you? This is what you have as a support system? This is what you have as a motivator?

"I have seen people inspired more by their enemies than some of the people they're confiding in"

I have been through people judging me based on the trial and error in my life, and I'm sure you have as well. But how else are we going to learn without trial and error? How else are we going to get familiar and comfortable in certain situations if we don't have trial and error? And how are we going to know who is in our corner if we don't go through this process? The trial and error in your life should give you the indication of who you can trust. This should create truth that only comes with going through something.

There have been so many times and situations that have brought on "trial and error," but have also brought on an answer about the people in your life as well. It should give you a sense of comfort that you now know who they are. It should give you a sense of comfort to know that you don't have to deal with them anymore. They weren't in your corner anyway! It was only through your trial and error that you now realize that they never had anything good to say about you in the first place. It was only through your trial and error that you realize that they have always been wishing the worse on you. Why? Because you have something they want. Maybe it's the way you look and carry yourself that they are jealous of. Maybe it's your personality! The way that people flock to you that has them irritated because when you come around you become the center of attention. Or maybe it's your ability to handle things that come your way that bothers them. They wish they could handle things better.

You thought that you were amongst friends. But you aren't! They were only around you because they were benefiting from your energy and charisma. And now that it is time for them to help carry the burden in your life, they would rather tear you down because they don't know anything else. They were hanging with you to mask their ability. And now that you have taken a wrong turn in life they don't know how to help you make the right one. Instead they keep holding their foot on the gas as you go off the cliff. But then you find yourself. Somewhere along the line the clouds split to allow the sun to comfort you. You realize that it is not as bad as you once thought and the storm has now given way to sunshine and a rainbow. God has shown you a way through his promise to man that he has always been there for you.

In the meantime, the people who you thought were in your corner are trying to make their way back into your fold. You remember when they weren't so willing to be there for you while you were going through the "Perfect Storm" in your life. You remember when they were taking cover as the waves got bigger with each complaint and criticism. You remember when they were adding their two cents to a check they thought you would never be able to cash. But they had it all wrong because during the perfect storm in your life they didn't take into account why they were around you in the first place. They didn't take into account why they enjoyed being in your presence.

"Your struggles have shown the weakness in them while showing you the strength in yourself."

You can't even believe that they ever doubted you or your ability. You can't believe that they didn't know you after all this time. But they didn't know you. They knew that you were who you said you were and how you presented yourself. You just didn't know them. You didn't know that all this time they were using you to keep their spirits up about themselves. You didn't know that all this time they have been piggy backing off all the things that made them see themselves through you. So every time you failed at something they feel that they have failed just the same. Every time things went wrong with you, they felt like it had tainted them in some way. I couldn't tell you where it comes from, this selfishness, but what I do know is that you better start seeing the people in your life for who they are.

They will always be judgmental and unsympathetic. They will always be supportive in success and damaging when you're unsuccessful. They will be unassuming and unyielding when they feel that they have to tear down your position to validate their own. Even when they don't have to be so brutal they will be because they don't know how to be reasonable to your struggle. They don't know how to have empathy for your desire to want and need an answer to your decision making skills.

Once again, they aren't taking into account that you put yourself out there to get hurt while everything in their life has been careful and calculated. They aren't taking into account that you want to live more by your desires than the rules and regulations of cautious people. They hate that they can't be more of a risk taker like you. They hate that they can't get over the butterfly affect every time they have to make a conscious choice on desire more than the advice taken from other people. They envy you so much that it plays on their psyche about themselves. They envy you so much that they hate the fact that they can't get over the unconscious weight they carry because of your willingness to put yourself in harm's way.

"All the positives about you have brought out all the negatives about them."

All the positive things people see in you have brought on all the negative things people see about them. And every chance they get they are going to make you look like you can't handle the "trial and error" in your life. Once again, every chance they get they are going to make it seem as though you have been riding their coat tails and not the other way around. Every chance they get they are going to make it seem like they have been the life of the party all this time. They just haven't been given a chance to prove themselves with you around. But your "trial and error" was designed to ground you so that God could protect you while everyone around you was taking shots at you. How else could God get your attention?

How else could he make his case with you about him, if he didn't make his case with you about them?

God knew that you would come to your senses about the people around you, eventually. God knew that you were never going to listen until he let you go through these hardships in your life. He knows your desire to live. He knows your desire to love. He knows your desire to fit in. He evens knows your desire to be acknowledged by your friends and family. God just wanted to show you who was worthy of that. He wanted to show you through your free will who was worthy of being around such a SPECIAL person like yourself. You have been honest and straightforward all your life. You have just been honest and straightforward with the wrong people. God knows that you want to do right. He knows that you feel like….

"If I can only get it right this time"

I would be fine. But you wouldn't be fine because while you're trying to get it right about yourself the people around you are trying to get what they said about you right as well. They don't want to be wrong about what they said about you. They're steady trying to make their point about you without looking like they're jealous or bitter. Even when you have made your point with your family and friends, they are still waiting for the moment when their arguments are going to be made about your decision making skills. They feel like it's only a matter of time before the man you chose is going to make their case for them. One thing that I have always been fascinated about when it comes to women and men—is how long they take to get to the desire part of themselves after going through trial and error. I would think that you would be tired of not only questioning everything in your lives, but having everyone else question those things as well. I would think that after dealing with the negatives of everybody's complaints and criticism about your decision making skills, you would be motivated to move on to the next thing and make all of the naysayers eat their words.

However, that's not the case! I can't understand the time that is wasted after the trial and error has worn off. If anybody deserves the right to move on and have something work out for them, it's *you*. If anybody deserves the right to tell family and friends they need to shut up and allow you to figure it out, it's you. This whole time we as men and women have allowed family and friends the argument that a new relationship will never make it, simply because they haven't gotten over the trial and error part of your life. Isn't it ironic? After all, they know you better than you know yourself, from what you keep telling everybody. So how could they be wrong about you? You have made their case for them because you have not accepted the trial and error in your life for what it was. But I am here to tell you that…

"The hardest thing for us to do is accept the trial and error in our lives… and move on."

This whole time you as men and women have known what you are and were capable of. And yet, you continue to allow the people around you and society to hold you hostage with your history. You moved on a long time ago, therefore, why are you even allowing them to bring it up? Why are you allowing them to keep you in the moments of your past? They have even made it seem like it is a good thing for you to go back into your past and hold onto your trial and error as a blueprint to why you should be more cautious now. But what you should be using your trial and error for is memories on how you no longer chose to be held hostage by that history. You should be using this as a reminder that you are better than what you have settled for in other people's opinions and doubts about you. You should be using it as a motivation to laugh at your critics, as you make your way beyond their thoughts and opinions about you. You have the ability to deal with any and every situation that is thrown your way. But somewhere along the line you have allowed this trickle-down effect to be a part of your makeup when dealing with the people in your life.

Yes! You have made a mess of your life and getting back to square one has become a daunting task, especially now that you haven't allowed the people in your life to keep you down with your trial and error. You don't have their best interest at heart anymore. And why should you? They have not earned the right to give you their opinions about how you're going to get back on the upside of your life. They have not earned the right to even be in your presence as it stands—because they were the first to jump on the bandwagon of your misery. But with that being said, "You go girl… I mean… really go." And "You go, boy…. I mean…. really go". Go on about your life and get what you have always deserved before the skeptics came along. And what you deserve is a man who appreciates you for taking a chance on him. What you deserve is a woman who appreciates you for showing her that you're ready to silence the critics.

Let the world know that you're not going to be held hostage by your trial and error. Get back to having a good time in life and show the people in your life that you are going to live your life to the fullest. Show your family and friends that they made a mistake when they doubted your abilities to mask over their own. You are usually a happy person, but since you start listening to every Tom, Dick and Harry about your situation, you have lost that element of yourself. But you can't do that! You can't lose yourself in order for them to find themselves. You can't lose your case about yourself to make their case for them. If you let them tell it you are headed for a disaster because nothing about your past has shown them that you know how to do anything else but ruin everything you come in contact with. How could you? You haven't been successful at anything. But you have—you've been extremely successful!

"You have been extremely successful at ruining your life."

So if you've been extremely successful at ruining your life, can't you be extremely successful at changing it? You haven't failed at anything that you have put your mind to. And knowing this should not only put you at ease but give you a sense of worth that was always there for you to benefit from. This is not something that God created in you today. He was just giving you a moment to find it. And now that you've found it, what are you going to do with it? It's always been in you. Now you just have to tap into it and use it for your greater good instead of your demise. We all know that it is so easy to get ourselves in trouble or make a bad decision on something or someone. But the greater reward comes in knowing that not only did you sacrifice for your desire but that it worked out for you.

There is no greater feeling than getting something right. I will even go further and say that there is no greater feeling than putting yourself in harm's way and getting it right because it will not only silence your critics but bring on a joyful noise that only comes with loving someone and having them love you back. You have the right to love and to be loved. And the only way you're going to know its existence is to take the trial and error in your life and use it to your advantage. Know that you have given the people in your life enough excuses and reasons to last them a lifetime and move on. There is a man or a woman waiting for you to show them that your trial and error have made you a better person so they can benefit from it.

CHAPTER 7

Make a Move or Make a Decision

Oftentimes, in the dating scene and life for that matter, there comes a time when a drastic decision or move has to be made in order to see if things are going to work. I refer to this as the **"black and white"** way of doing things. This way of doing things is very rare in a society filled to the brim with a lot of grey areas. I am actually one of those people who prefer the black and white way of doing things because it makes it easier for me to balance two sides of my life, instead of not knowing how many sides I would have to balance by allowing some grey area. I prefer knowing what the ramifications are going to be for using a simple approach rather than being all over the board not knowing what the consequences are going to be for using society's approach of making excuses for all the angles that they are coming from. However, try explaining this to my friends who have always told me that I take things too literal. And when it comes to the getting to know process, I feel there should be no grey area if you're trying to balance out your lives together and understand exactly where things are.

So many times we are afraid to make a move or a decision surrounding a relationship that we want because we think that we may miss out on something better. In turn, we do what most people do when they are too frightened to make a move or decision—we live by the word, *because*. We live by our excuses and reasons about that other person that stop us from making a move or making a decision. Some of us have even made a name for those reasons and excuses called **"red flags"**.

We think that anytime a person challenges us to see things differently than what we're used to—that's a red flag that tells us that this person is not worth making a move or a decision on, But that is exactly who you should be making a move or a decision on because they are preparing you for future events with them. They are preparing you to know their family and friends. They are preparing you to go to church functions and job outings. But many of us think that they are being pushy and combative because we've never had anyone in our lives who cared as much. We don't even know the difference between a good reason or a bad excuse when it comes to being challenged to be better men and women. That is why we justify our reasons and excuses for not making a move or a decision on the "because."

"Well... I didn't like him because! And I didn't want to be with her because!"

If you find someone using **"because"** to justify their reasons for not making a move or a decision with regard to being with someone, it generally means that the person is afraid to do so. Typically, it's the person who didn't want to open up to the possibility of something that is the one who was afraid to make a move or a decision. The **"because"** became the red flag or their way out more than anything the other party did or didn't do. So many times we set ourselves up for failure because we wait for our potential mate to make a move or a decision for us rather than be aggressive with our desire to make it happen. The reason for this is we don't want to be held responsible if things don't go according to plan. However, an unhealthy premature decision that is not actually a decision but more like a *"let's see what happens"* doesn't subject you to ridicule because you're not actually making the decision or move more than just going along with it. I am not actually buying the cow more than I am just renting it. So the question now becomes...

"Why should I buy the cow when I can get the milk for free?"

Why should I make a move or a decision on a man or a woman to be in a relationship when I am getting all the perks that go with being in a relationship, in the getting to know process? Men don't generally create this situation. As I mentioned in the first chapter, men typically go with the flow while they wait for women to tell them how things are going to play out. Therefore, making any premature decisions with a woman they don't know is not in a man's makeup. I have also noticed at times that we as men and women will make the things we can't control an excuse not to make a move or a decision. We make things that have nothing to do with making a move or a decision the reason as to why we're not making one. But that's not a good reason—that's a bad excuse. And it will never get better as long as we continue to take each other on this merry-go-round in life trying to figure out if we are going to get the ultimate prize that is each other.

For the most part, as men we know that you kind of like us because why else would you be spending time with us and allow us to spend time with you. That is why it is confusing for us sometimes because we don't know where we stand in the grand scheme of things. The one thing men do know is we're going to sit back and wait for women to make a move or decision on us. Women think time is going to help them make a move or decision on men, but time never stops. Even if a woman does wait the necessary time to justify why she is making a move or decision on a man, that still doesn't necessarily mean that she will. We as a society make being in a relationship or making a move or decision on one, about time, when there have been women who have taken a chance on men—way before time would have permitted.

Like, one day it dawned on me while I was spending time with my girl that she didn't wait on time to help her make a move or a decision on me. Instead, it was her interaction with me and how comfortable she was in assigning me that role—that became the determining factor. Of course, it doesn't work this way for everyone, because most men are not ready for that position, even if he is ready for the rights to it. And the reason why they are not ready is because they have not been prepped or trained to carry out the responsibility of standing in that role. But I would be remiss if I didn't bring up the fact that there are good and bad reasons for making a move or decision on a man right away. But I know why women take such a long time making a move or making a decision on a man.

On one side, women don't make a move or decision on a man so quickly because you have to justify to society why you are doing so when you barely know him. Plus, you're not sure if you want a man to have the same rights as you to demand out of you something that you're not ready for. So you don't push the envelope even though it would make the transition from meet and greet to the relationship much smoother. And on the other side, you have listened to everyone and everything tell you that time will dictate that decision for you, not realizing that your desire and his ability to meet your desires should dictate that. A man will never be comfortable with making a move or a decision when he doesn't know for sure that he is familiar with all of your ways of wanting things done because contrary to popular belief…

"Men are not afraid of commitment! They are afraid of change."

Men are not afraid of being the man that you've always wanted. He's wondering if you have told him everything about you and your desires before he allows you to make a move or decision on your life and his. Men are asking themselves "Has she been totally honest with me about her desires and how she wants things done on a regular basis?" He's steady asking himself is this the routine that we're going to have for the long haul or are there going to be a couple of wrinkles in there at some point? Even when we as men are not making the move or decision to go further into a relationship with women, we need to know that your desires and demands are not going to take away our individuality all together. We as men need to feel that women are not going to take away everything about us and replace it with everything about you.

That is why the back and forth games that your emotions present at times has us on pins and needles! If we knew that the things that you asked us for at the start were never going to change, then our demeanor towards those things wouldn't either. It is a very simple process that most women continue to make difficult with your rules and regulations because your true feelings won't let you go there. Society and the people around you have told you that it is too soon. You couldn't possibly be ready to make a move or decision on this man after only a few interactions. What about the three months that you are supposed to make him wait before he even gets a little taste of your true emotions for him? But who is playing the game now?

What about your mom who doesn't like him? What about your children who are uncomfortable about you meeting someone because you haven't been with anybody since their dad? Or what about all the books you have read that told you it would never work out if you take things too fast? This whole time you have been listening to everyone tell you what's best for you and you wonder why he is just as confused about his position in your life as you are of yours in his. You don't know which way to go with your mind or your emotions. You haven't even allowed him to do the little things in your life so that he could make somewhat of a case against the onslaught that you're taking from everyone around you. They have made you complacent about your desire to make a move or a decision on him while you struggle to make sense of it all.

In the meantime, the life is being sucked out of his desire to continue waiting for you to show him that you believe he's the one. You keep claiming that you want him! But at what cost are you willing to suffer to make your point and his? You're treating this decision like it's the most drastic decision you're going to make or have made in your life. You're treating this move as though it will be the most damaging thing you've ever done. You can't even see that you are making it more and more difficult by going back and forth. You don't realize how not making a move or decision is not only playing on your psyche, but his as well, because he feels like if you don't trust yourself to make a move or a decision on him then why should he trust himself to make a move or decision on you.

There are so many men out there who feel that they have made their case for women to make a move or decision on them. So why is she taking so long? Why is she not getting the point that I am trying to build a LIFE with her? Why is she not getting the point that she is the woman that I have been looking for all my life, even if it took me only a moment to know? You are spending so much time worrying about how things are going to turn out in the move or decision instead of making one and seeing how things are going to turn out. You are spending time trying to make sure that the decision or move you're trying to make is going to work instead of getting yourself into it so that you can get your answer once and for all.

"But you don't want a good man! You want a good situation."

You're trying to make sure that when you do make a move or a decision that all the stars are going to be aligned. Not understanding that the more you bring imbalanced emotions and decisions to the table, the more imbalanced his responsibility to you is going to be as well. You're worrying so much about what your girlfriends and society is going to say if you don't do things according to their standards. Society and the people in your life are scared of the possibility that love can make its way into your presence naturally. Doubt has set the tone in your life instead of you. And skepticism has followed suit. You spend your days fighting mentally and emotionally amongst yourself. And you're always looking for everybody else's answers and decisions about what you should do because...

"The thought of being wrong is worst than the feeling of being right."

You know that making a move or decision on a man has a greater possibility of not being successful more than the potentials of being successful. But I am here to say that you can and should relish in those "I told you so" moments because you have the right to. You have been looking for this kind of man all your life. You have been looking for this kind of love and respect all your life. And now that it is right there for the taking, you let the people around you make that move or decision for you. You let the people in your life take the wind out of your sails with their way of doing things and how they make moves or decisions on their potential mates. But you're better than that! You are better than what they settle for in their decision making skills. You are even better than what you settle for in your own way of thinking.

I don't understand how we as men and women don't relish in our *"I told you so"* moment in our lives, but we let everybody else relish in their *"I told you so"* moments in our lives. And all the while you've got a good man on hold, waiting to embrace his position in your life. But he can't take on that position until you give it to him. The longer you wait for a good situation, the longer it's going to take for a good man to find his way into your life. The longer you wait on your girlfriends or society to tell you that it's okay for you to take a chance on "Mr. Right," it will become evident that he doesn't want to be anything beyond Mr. Right now. But your friends have told you that if he can't wait for you, then he's not worth it. But what your friends and society forgot to tell you is he stopped caring about wait-ing on you a long time ago because even though you haven't made a move on him or a decision about him, you haven't let him in on any plans to do so anytime soon. It's like having a band wait around to see if they are going to play at a concert that they were never booked for. All he wants to know is that you will let him know about your plans to go forward with him real soon, and giving him something to look forward to every time he sees you is not a bad idea either.

Now I'm sure that there are those of you who are asking, "What if I make a move or a decision on a man too soon?" My answer to that would be is whoever picked three months as the ideal time to make a person wait for you to make a move or a decision is really telling you that you don't have the ability to discern between a man who is capable and a man who is not; or that you have time to waste. This is not an attack on books that are trying to give a good perspective! I just have to question the common sense that goes into it. And for those of you who have made a quick decision on a man or a woman and it didn't work out, I would say that you should be thankful that it didn't take you three months to find out that he or she was not worth wasting any more of your valuable time. Ask yourself how many times did you take it slow with a man or a woman and it didn't work out? What is your excuse then? Why is it considered to be wrong when you make a move or a decision quickly and it doesn't work out? But when you take your time making a move or a decision, is it not considered in the same way?

I have made a move and decision both ways and they didn't work out. That doesn't mean that one way should take more credit for working any more than the other way should take the blame for not working. It doesn't mean that I'm going to always fail at one way of making a move or a decision more than the other way, and vice versa! And just for the records, ladies… it's not the waiting that men find disturbing. It's the waiting with no end in sight or an indication of an end in sight that men take the most issue with. We would rather a woman make a move or a decision with regard to not seeing us—rather than to have us go back and forth, not knowing when she is going to finally make one. But this is what has happened when I look at the fact that I can have my cake and eat it too. And that's not just men that I'm talking about. The whole world has been made available to us. So making a move or a decision and settling for just one man or woman has become a daunting task, indeed.

"Nobody wants to live with the consequences of choosing wrong more than the reward of choosing right."

As women, you are trying to get closer to your desire to find love and have it find you. But all the while you're sitting in the wings waiting for it to make a good case while you continue to make a bad decision about it. Therefore, you may find yourself questioning: "How is it that some people can just make that decision and it just works for them?" All the while, it appears that every man or woman who comes your way is like a temp job who has no desire to hire you once the honeymoon period is over.

But it all goes back to the first chapter when I described women as the wireless router and the man as a computer. He can only connect to your way of doing things when you present him with the signal that is going to give him the indication that he won't be shut down when he decides to oblige. So how bad do you want it? It doesn't seem like you want it as much as you say, because you continue to listen to all the outside elements and influences that will never render a result that you will be satisfied with. You're living by everyone else's desires for you as a potential mate. They see that you have a man waiting for an answer. But they don't care because…

"They would rather be right about your misery than wrong about your happiness."

The people in your life would rather see you struggling than succeeding because they know that being wrong would make them look more like a person who didn't have your best interest at heart instead of a supporter. It would make them look more like their way of thinking matters more than yours because you have allowed them to play a vital part in something that they shouldn't be given a right to take a part in. But it's not just them! It's the book that you are currently reading from an author who gets paid to host comedy shows and awards ceremonies. You've even confided in the girl who does your hair every Tuesday who filled you in on the fact that she read the same book, and having a name that is common is better than having sense that is more common. And yes, everyone is entitled to their opinion.

"But they shouldn't have an opinion that allows them to take away your right to make a move or decision."

Their opinion should not become the validation you claim to need in order to make a move or a decision on the love that has been eluding you all of your life. I'm not even asking you to take my opinion into account either. All I am saying is that at the end of the day, your life is going to be filled with happiness or misery because you created that situation—even though everyone around you gave their two cents on how you should be doing it. And rather you like it or not, you are still going to be held responsible for how it turns out. So you might as well be the person making the move or decision. Time is not going to determine whether "Mr. Man" is going to work out or not. Your interactions and ability to get your needs met is going to do that. And if he shows you that he is able to meet your needs immediately, then he should benefit just as quickly.

Stop letting the people in your life subject you to their way of making a move or decision and start taking it upon yourself to bring your way to the table. Start relishing in your own *"I told you so"* moments instead of letting them play friend-turned- psychiatrist every time you find a man who is thinking about making a move or decision on you. Stop reading the books of people presenting concepts which take away the logic in your reasons to take a chance on love and start enjoying the process that comes with wanting to know if a man is going to work out. Stop allowing your girlfriends to put you in a frame of mind that has you questioning the motives of your desires for a man and start showing them that you're going to be comfortable with your move or decision when the opportunity presents itself.

I would imagine that it is quite frustrating given all of the things that you have to take into account just to make a move or decision. It must be exhausting to juggle all the emotions and opinions. It must be heartbreaking because you know that he's out there, but you feel that time is running out in your search to find him. You know that it can't be you, but you just can't seem to turn off the voices and opinions because they mean too much to you right now while you struggle with reason. Their voices and opinions mean too much to you while struggle with your desire to know if a man is going to work out for you. I know that you would be magnificent in love's presence if you just went on and made the move or decision on it. I know that you would be the talk of town if you just let it naturally consume you. I know that you would be okay if you would just throw yourself at the mercy of it.

So when are you going to take control of your life and leave all the naysayers behind? When are you going to see life for yourself the way you interpret it? You haven't been that same woman that you've been in the past. You took a chance on your business ventures and now you're a serious businesswoman. You didn't take anyone's advice on making a move or a decision when it was time to secure your life financially. So why all of a sudden when it's time to make a decision on the man that has been waiting for you since you were an intern at your law firm, do you now have cold feet? You have been dating him for three months now and you're not sure that you want to change how things are because you're afraid that it might ruin how things have been. That is when you bring your one girlfriend to the table who doesn't like him because he didn't go out of his way to appease her while being with you.

It seems like to me that you need the people in your life around for sabotaging purposes so you can have someone agreeing with your reasons for being stagnate. You have made a mockery of this man's time. And you wonder why he is a little on edge with you. Your reasons for not making a move or decision have become more about control than time. The time that you claimed to set aside to get to know him has expired. You want to make a move on him or a decision about him but you're not sure when because somewhere in your mind you have painted a picture that has you holding your heart hostage. **FEAR** has overstepped its boundaries and has become the daily dose of excuse serum you need to keep your so-called future love at bay. The saddest thing about this is you don't want him to make the decision for you because from the way things have been going lately you know that you would probably be looking for someone else to go to dinner and your favorite tear jerker movie with.

"You don't like him enough to say yes, but you don't dislike him enough to say no."

You go back to the resources which stopped you from being in something serious in the first place—namely, your friends! They will surely hold you up in your decision to not make one because they were responsible for the state you are currently in. They are extremely motivated to validate their reasons for sabotaging your potential involvement with him, even though love has made no attempt to be in their life since cartoons were in black and white. Yes! Misery loves company. And more than that it loves being right because misery doesn't have to apologize for being wrong. Your friends know that they can always revert back to blaming you because it's your life and you're the one who is supposed to be making the final decision anyway. Better you than them, right! So you thought! Your mind is growing tired with the fact that you have to make a move or decision soon. It's been two months, thirty days and twenty three hours. What are you waiting on? You care more about the ridicule more than your sanity. And making the wrong move or decision now is going to really make you seem like you have no clue as to what you're doing. But I am here to say that….

"The only way that you can recognize BS is to open yourself up to it."

When you're not making a move or decision, how can you call a man's bluff? How can you know what he is capable of? How can you know if he is going to live up to what he is telling you? And why should you be waiting three months for him to come with that fact? Why shouldn't you be telling yourself that you need an answer now? The longer it takes for you to open up, the longer it is going to take for you to get an answer. The longer it takes for you to throw down a rope, the longer it is going to take for him to start climbing. You're trying to soften the blow of making a move or decision rather than make one and live with the results because you think that it's going to ruin the other relationships in your life.

You may defend, "it has taken me a long time to build this relationship with my girls! And you just want me to throw it all away over some guy I just met two months, thirty days and twenty three hours ago? Depending on the month?" No! That's not what I am saying at all. What I am saying is… the longer you take to make a move or a decision about the guy you're dating, the longer it's going to take for you to make your case with your girls that you are and were capable of getting it right. The longer you take to make a move or decision with him, the longer it is going to take to see his potentials and how those things fall in line with your desires.

All men are asking for is an opportunity to prove themselves. And it's not going to do him any good if he has to sit around and wait for you to get your act together so he can present you with his case. You want to know anyway? Don't you? You want to know if he is a feast or famine kind of guy who is going to make all of your dreams come true or all of your nightmares appear. And just for the records, ladies…you don't want a man who caters to your family to make his point more than catering to you. You don't want that kind of man in your life because he will make it about them more than you, while trying to prove his point about himself. There is nothing worse than having your family like the man you're with more than you. So you better make a move or a decision about him before he makes a move or decision about them—especially if you have an overbearing family who feels as though they should benefit from your mate more than you.

And with that being said, let me ask you—what's stopping you from making a move or decision on the guy you're seeing? What is stopping you from making a move or decision on him when he has shown you that he has the capacity and capability to meet your needs? And why are you letting your family and friends dictate that more than you? You got what you've always asked for in a man. Making him wait any longer to prove himself is only going to have you waiting longer to have your answer. So make that move or decision so you can either move on with him or find the man that you have been looking for all of your life. Otherwise, you're going to fall into the trap that most women have fallen into by telling themselves that….

GOOD THINGS COME TO THOSE WHO WAIT!

But good things come to those who are waiting on what? Jesus Christ to come back? Now this is an interesting concept because I've always heard men and women say that when you don't look for a man or a woman, you find one. And when you do look for one, it never comes. Well, I'm hear to tell you that if you thought this way about finding a job you would be **BROKE**! I mean! I wonder whoever came up with this concept anyway. And what were they going through in their life at the time that they would say such a thing? I'm almost guaranteed that it had nothing to do with finding a mate. Oftentimes, when you're not proactive as a human being, good things don't usually find you. As a matter of fact! There is a greater potential for you to find anything but. When you're not putting forth an effort to find a mate, the percentages of you finding love or love finding you is little to none.

Once again, society has given us this false sense that our effort won't be appreciated or needed. So we enter the getting to know process not giving the effort that is required to authentically sustain getting to a relationship status. I know men and women who have lived their whole lives on this very concept. And they wonder why the relationship never evolved into anything. So they go looking for a man or woman to convince them that their energy will make up for the fact that your energy is lacking to make things work. So you both go into the get to know process waiting for the other person to make a drastic move towards showing each other that you're serious about being together. Unfortunately, a lot of time is often wasted in this process. That's why I would not recommend waiting for anything. Go and make it happen because one of the most difficult things to witness is the person you wanted to be with, being with someone else—because you decided to wait.

CHAPTER 8

Identity Crisis

When I look at the world today, I have mixed emotions and thoughts about men and women as you can see from the first few chapters of my book. I don't mind accepting the fact that I have taken a very aggressive stand on those things that I see men and women struggling with. But none of the things that I mentioned thus far could be more disappointing to me than the identity crisis that we have created in the last twenty years as men and women. Since the test of time we have been given somewhat of a blueprint to go on in order for things to take on a very natural course. And even though we as men and women have steered away from some of those beliefs and rules, the original application still applies in order for those things to work. When I think about what that application is the one word that comes to mind is "accountability." We have been a society that has become extremely unaccountable for each other and ourselves. We are going through what I call an "identity crisis." Our beliefs have changed. Our morals have changed. And last but not least—our times have changed. But all is not lost in translation. There is an old saying that...

"If you don't stand for something, you will fall for anything."

I will be the first to say that I was one of those people who had fallen, and had fallen far! I, like most men and women, had gotten myself caught up in a societal flow that didn't render me God's interpretation of myself. I was limiting myself to an interpretation created by others to define me as a man and my position in a woman's life, and I'm not alone. There are those of you out there who are not only allowing a society to render you their interpretation of you as a man, but you're not even defending yourselves to say that you're not going to allow this blatant disregard of your position to continue to exist. That you're not going to take this lack of respect lying down. But you have accepted it, even though you have had the ability all this time to change it. So if you're not going to fight for your right to be seen in the correct light, how are women ever going to see you that way? You are so much more of a man than that. God did not make you in his image to be limited. So why are you allowing these limitations to be put on you as a man?

You absolutely know that your position has been taken for granted, and yet you worry about a society who is still going to make you take responsibility for the fact that you have not lived up to your true potentials. As a man, you have lost your total perspective on your boundaries and what you have allowed to define you. Who have you been all of your life—because you certainly haven't been you? You think that you are amongst friends, but you're not! You've laid down with the enemy without question or discernment, skepticism or restraint when you should have been keeping your guards up. Women definitely have their guards up when dealing with you. And yet, you continue to cater to every woman you meet, allowing them to over-look the strength in you so that it can make a case for themselves. They have you fight an uphill battle with yourself and the people around you. But I am here to say that you don't have to sit back and allow these labels to be placed on you anymore.

There are many women who are saying that they're not help-ing any man live up to God's interpretation of himself. And as men, this is the approach that you're catering to? This is the approach you have allowed women to sell you on? You couldn't have given yourself a worse thing to agree with them on. That is why I asked you in the previous chapter not to take a chance on any woman who is not will-ing to help you live up to your potentials so she could BENEFIT. Why should you adhere to your calling as a man when that calling is not only being misinterpreted, but also disrespected?

This is the sole reason why most situations are doomed before they start because God's interpretation is being constantly pushed to the back burner. This claim is validated in the independent approach that most women have decided to come at men with. Not only are you a man without limitations, but you should never be with a woman who validates herself by an interpretation which limits you as a man. You should never be with a woman who has forgotten or doesn't know that she is degrading and disrespecting your position as a man in order to validate her position as a woman. And shame on us as men that we have allowed that.

We have allowed the women of today to use a calling that was meant for us to be transparent when dealing with them. We have sat in the backgrounds and have allowed this crisis to become a part of our make-up as men. When are you going to say enough is enough? And that your existence is based on God's interpretation of you as a man and not everyone else? It's funny how we would go out of our way to defend ourselves against any other man who disrespects us in our position. But when it comes to women, we have allowed them to interpret their belief system and not so much as a challenge has gone their way. Why have we become so complacent in this process?

I have to go out on a limb and say that as a man I have not always lived up to God's interpretation or my potentials, and there are many of you in the world who have not lived up to their potential as well. However, that doesn't mean that you have to stay lost just because you have been lost. You don't have to be a part of the problem all of your life just because you have been a problem for most of it. Let society tell it, you've been a failure all of your life and there's no way that you're up for changing. There is no way that you're going to come out and defend yourself because they can always go back to when you weren't such a great guy with potential, if you had any at all.

That will be a woman's way of trying to sabotage your future because their arrogance have told them that if you couldn't amount to anything with them, than there's no possible way that you're going to amount to anything with anyone else. And society has jumped on their bandwagon and joined in their pity party about you. Society has convinced them that you will never live up to God's interpretation because you couldn't even live up to theirs. Society has made these women feel like their interpretation of you matters more than God's. But it doesn't and it never will.

You were a man when the doctor told your mother and father what you were going to be in the embryo stage. So feeling like you have to convince men or women on what you are as a man is not your job because God has already validated you. Before all of the trophies, accomplishments, rewards, acknowledgements, mistakes and bad decisions, you were a man. And now that you have had to do some growing up, you are still the same man that you were when you weren't being validated by those things. God's interpretation of you as a man has not changed even though the perceptions of the people around you, have. So you need to start concentrating your effort and energy towards God's interpretation because that matters more than anything society could ever try to put on you. And knowing this should not only put you at ease but give you such a sense of worth that you should have no problem defending God's interpretation. Here it is... we as men and women are going at people with an individual mentality trying to sell them on a relationship concept, and we wonder why things are so messed up.

The reason why we don't use God's interpretation is because we know that in the long run we will not have an argument otherwise. A man treating a woman by God's interpretation of herself will totally take away a mentality that has no excuse. As men, we have the ability to be everything a woman needs us to be. We just need to make some changes in our approach and make up in order to tap into it. But because you are so worried about a woman using the things in your past to justify her not acknowledging you for what you are now, you take the easy way out. But all you have to do is hang in there to show her that you have always had the ability to handle things.

Instead you take the easy way out because you want an instant gratification for making the changes necessary for women to trust you again. But as men, you have to start understanding that it is going to take even longer to get your point across after all the men these women have been dealing with that wasn't living up to God's interpretation. Most women don't understand that it is only going to hurt them in the long run that you're not living up to God's interpretation. And at this point, women really don't care. Especially those women who haven't lived up to God's interpretation much in their own lives! My mom used to tell me that...

"Women apply everything to themselves"

when it comes to men and women. So there is no way you are not ashamed that you have not lived up to God's interpretation, if she is ashamed that she hasn't lived up to it in her life. You're no better than her if you let her tell it. There is no possible way that you can change when she is not ready to change. There is no way that you can be successful when she doesn't feel like she can be successful. That's why she tries to keep you in your past. That's why she tries to keep you remembering when she was cheated on, and when her ex dogged her because she feels that until she can let go of her past, she will never allow you to let go of yours. Even when you tried to tell her that her girlfriends were the reason for her current situation with men, she wasn't listening to you. But you have to tell yourself that you are going to be the telling factor in your relationship even if she doesn't believe you.

There are some women that are limiting men to an interpretation that God never intended for men to have. And all your female counterparts who have wrote books and songs giving you this misleading interpretation, knows this. Of course, they have profited from your ignorance while most of them have gone on and found a man who doesn't allow them to take away their true identity while you struggle to find even one man to take some kind of initiative with you. One minute it's *"I'm an independent woman"* and the next minute it's **"Can you pay my bills?"** And you wonder why men are sitting in the wings waiting to see what other bandwagon you're going to jump on next. And men, we are no better, because we only thought that this "independent woman" thing was for entertainment purposes. We never thought that this interpretation would get so out of hand. We just thought that it would pass on by like all the other fads women created throughout the years.

I am confident that most women—at least the *real* women—trusted that men would stand up and offer a powerful response to the New Age woman when she emerged. But once women realized that we as men were not responding with a powerful response or backlash, the idea that they could take a man's position for granted and play victim in that spread like a virus. The interpretation of just being an "independent" woman wasn't enough for some women anymore. They wanted more. So they decided that it was time to take over God's interpretation of you as a man and make it their own. They knew you wouldn't say anything because they could always bring up your past to make their point as to why they have had to become you. Why they have had to become more responsible for themselves. But I am here to say that...

"The only women who continue to dwell on your past, is those women who are not thinking about a future."

And you let them off the hook because never once did they take on God's interpretation of themselves to help you understand God's interpretation of yourself. Never once did you question or challenge them to live up to God's interpretation of themselves so that they could help you live up to God's interpretation of you. I mean... still to this day man carries the largest burden on this earth. And yet, women get to take all of the credit while you take all of the blame. But if you know as a man that you're going to take the blame for not living up to God's interpretation of yourself as a man— you might as well fight for it. Right! I mean.... what has become of men that you continue to carry the largest burden on this earth while allowing this misinterpretation? Why have you allowed for society to dictate your worth based on some woman's experiences with you and not God's interpretation? Why have you allowed society to dictate your worth based on everything else but what God says about you? That's why Jesus Christ says that...

"He who is without sin cast the first stone."

You have allowed yourselves to be stoned to death in the last twenty five years. You have allowed women and society to cast a negative shadow over you that has been looming for the last twenty years and not so much as an argument has made its way into their presence. So when are you going to stand up and accept God correcting you and adhering to your responsibility as a man? When are you going to shake off society's restraints and stop allowing them to put you into the grave before your time? You have a woman that is waiting for you to get your act together. Your children are waiting for you to get your act together. Your family is waiting for you to get your act together. She doesn't know who you are but God knows who she is and what her true desire is. You may not know your children, but they are waiting to know you. You may not know how to be in a family, but they want to know what it is like to be around you.

Instead, you have surrounded yourself with those people who have a lack of respect for God's interpretation of you. They don't believe in you. And why should they? Nothing about you has shown them that you're even a fighter. Nothing about you has shown them that you are somebody that they are proud to know. You continue to play out man's interpretation because you think that if you defend God's interpretation they won't want anything to do with you anymore. But no one ever turns away from the light when all they've seen is darkness. No one ever turns away from certainty when all they have seen is uncertainty. You have had the ability all of your life to move mountains. And yet, you have spent it making molehills. You have spent it continuously going back to your old ways because you have given up on the good in yourself. You have given up on the good in yourself because you think that society or the people around you will never acknowledge or appreciate it. But what you don't see is that your indiscretions are no more a part of your makeup than they are for anyone else. And believe me when I say this....

"As long as you continue to allow society and women to base your reality upon *their* experiences with you— you will never be able to fulfill God's interpretation of yourself as a man."

As a man, you have never lived up to the goals and dreams you have had since you were a child. You have never lived up to your true identity so you can silence your critics. But you have it in you to be the man that you've always wanted to be. You just can't be afraid of accepting the truth about where you have been all this time. I can honestly say that I am no longer afraid to fight for a position that has been rightfully mine from the beginning of time. I am no longer afraid of the illusions that have been established by society to make me look like I am a man who can never live up to my true identity because I know now that it never left me. I was the one who left my true identity behind. And I recommend that you men out there in the world do the same.

Your true identity is what you came into this world with. All the mistakes and mishaps you have made along the way are only influences from other things that have taken you away from your true make-up. You are not who society says you are. You are not even what the people around you say that you are. You are who God says you are. And the only way your true identity is going to become what everybody will see and know is you have to fight for it. Otherwise, no one will ever truly know the real man in you.

"I will never be able to call myself a real man without God's interpretation."

Just because people approach you with their interpretation of things, doesn't mean that you have to accept it as such. We as men have been taught the correct interpretation of things all of our lives. So why are you accepting this interpretation that most women and society are coming at us with? Why aren't you owning up to and protecting your true identity? These are the questions you need to start asking yourselves and coming with a definitive answer. Otherwise, women will never trust you with the position you deserve. Now before I get to the women in this chapter, I have to be fair and say that I know this will be a new thing for most of you to hear. I know that for the most part, some of you have not been told of this ignorance that is playing itself out in our society and your lives today. And you ask, "What ignorance is that, Tonee?" Unfortunately, it's the ignorance of not knowing that…

"What you inspire in a man, is what he is going to be good at."

If you inspire nothing in a man, then he will be good at nothing. If you encourage him to do nothing, then he will be good at nothing. If you motivate him to do nothing, then he will be good at nothing. If you're not feeding the ego of a man's purpose, then he will be good at nothing in your life. Oftentimes, when I have brought to a woman's attention the need for a man to have inspiration and motivation in the proper direction, I receive a strong "pushback" or resistance to what I'm saying because most women feel that they should not have to use their energy to help a man or even motivate one. But I am here to say that not challenging a man to live up to his true identity is only going to have him taking your true identity for granted. That is why it is essential for you, as a woman, to know what your true identity and desires are. If you don't believe that you deserve a man taking care of and meeting your needs, you will never open up or attract those men who are willing to do so. And I understand that….

"Women want to be swept off their feet…whereas men want to be kept on their toes."

There are those of you who feel that a man should automatically know what his true identity is before he makes his way into your life. There are those of you who feel that a man should automatically know how you want things done before you give him a right to do so. But I am here to say that a man would be capable of living up to his true potentials if he had a woman that was living up to her true identity. Men would relish the moment where he would have the right to show a woman his true identity, if a woman supported that approach with her own identity. I am rather surprised, even by some of the women in my own family, who have seen the correct interpretation of how women should be with men. And yet, they still chose to acknowledge this brain-damaged way of thinking that they're going to use their identities to benefit themselves while they struggle with men. They still chose based off their ignorance to acknowledge an approach that is in no way shape or form going to get their needs met.

Somewhere along the line your identity has taken a backseat to an approach that will have you doing things that your mom never did, and your grandmother never had to do. You may even find yourself asking, how did it ever become this way? How did the male gender become so unenthusiastic about relationships? How did men become so uninspired with regard to their position in our lives? And how did we not see that this was going to eventually become a problem that we were going to have to deal with as women? I am here to tell you that these questions will continue to have no answer because men are depending on you to show them your true identity in order for his true identity to evolve. They are counting on women for motivation and inspiration to live up to God's interpretation of themselves. Your ability to do this will have men showing the world and God that you are worthy of mentioning and making a life with. So you should want to be the reason for a man's success.

My mom knew all to well her place in my stepfather's life, to get him to a point where his true identity was going to be present for her at all times. She knew that her identity was going to allow his identity to mirror God's interpretation and not hers. She knew that as long as she understood her place in his life, he would know his place in God. And with that, allow me to ask: Do you know your place in

116

a man's life? Do you know what role you are to play in a man living up to God's interpretation instead of your own? Or are you one of those women who are sitting in the wings waiting for him to interpret on his own his position in your life? That's what men need to know! They need to know how important your position as a woman is to you because they will use that observation as the basis to know where they will stand as far as their position in your life.

There are so many women saying to man that they are not bringing their true identity to the table to help a man with his. Why should I? Society has sold them on the fact that they don't need a man to make things easier for them. So most women feel that there is no need to help a man live up to his true potentials! I have even had women ask me, *"what happens if I help him in living up to God's interpretation and it doesn't work out? I help him live up to God's interpretation of things and he leaves me high and dry, only to take his act elsewhere?"* My answer to that would be one that says that it is just as hard for a man to find the kind of woman who is willing to help them live up to his true identity. Therefore, leaving that type of woman behind is not an option for me or any other man. There is no way that we're leaving that kind of woman behind. Society has made you think that a man will leave you even though you are helping him live up to God's interpretation. However, that couldn't be further from the truth because once again...

"No one turns from the light when all they have seen is darkness."

No one ever turns from the certainties that come with living up to their true identity. Let me ask you women a question: If you knew that man was going to live up to his true identity in your life, would you be there to make sure that he did? Then why not have that approach going into the getting to know process in the first place? You continue to say that you want a good man in your life. However, nothing about your approach is telling you that you need to be a good woman in order for your wishes to come true.

I always hear women say how much they want a real man, and a responsible man; however, the minute they have to help with that interpretation, they sit back and let a man struggle because their interpretation of themselves doesn't give man the ability or the belief that they should. You don't realize that you are the one who is behind his living up to his true identity. You don't realize that you are the one who is dictating what his motivation is or will be when getting to know you. In essence, where's your ability to motivate and to inspire? You're too busy working three jobs in order to maintain your status as an independent woman, and you wonder why your energy and effort to inspire a man is so low. But I am here to say that….

"He doesn't need you to lead by example! He needs and wants to be inspired by you so he can lead by example."

The only reason why you're stuck working three jobs is because you haven't inspired a man to work one job. He has bought into the emotional side of you instead of getting you to buy into the logical side of him. Of course he doesn't stand his ground because he's worried about you labeling with a negative response instead of bringing what you claimed you wanted—a real man! But a real man knows when to cater, when to stand his ground and when to be stern with his true identity. And he will never bring his true identity to the table when he knows that you are going to shoot it down with your New Age way of doing things. Once again... it wasn't his intention to take you for granted before you gave him the blueprint and okay to do so. There is an old saying that...

"Much is required of those who have much!"

So who are you to expect someone else to bring their true identity to the table when you have not brought yours? Who are you to expect a man to be a man when your ability to be a woman supporting that interpretation is non-existent? There's nothing more exciting than having a woman who knows her true identity and knows how to inspire a man to live up to God's interpretation. That kind of woman will never have anything to worry about because she will have the man and God rendering their love and energy to her. Now for those of you who don't know your true identity, you have everything to worry about. You really do. You have everything to worry about because you will never know another human beings true identity when your identity is not presenting itself.

As a man who is very aware of his identity, I can always tell when a woman is ready to help a man live up to his true identity. She is the kind of woman who doesn't worry about the things that most women worry about. She is the kind of woman that doesn't have a lot of questions about a man's position because she knows that her position dictates that. She is the kind of woman who knows her place with God and man. Therefore, I ask—what kind of woman are you? Are you the kind of woman who needs the answers before you present your true identity? Or are you a woman who truly believes that as long as you bring your true identity to the table, that not only will the man acknowledge you for it, but God will also? As a man, I can honestly say that.....

"I would rather be wrong for doing something in my true identity, than to be right for doing something out of it."

Our true identity gives us the ability to have a clear mind and see things for what they really are. That's what women need from us as men! And as men, we have to be willing to show them that our true identities are not going to take a back seat to their identities, if they want things to work out.

"A man will never take you serious as long as you continue to take his true identity for granted."

And he shouldn't take you serious. He shouldn't be willing to sacrifice who he really is to please you. And at the end of the day, you wouldn't appreciate it anyway! As men, you have adopted a woman's interpretation and society's interpretation of things more than God's interpretation and you wonder why everyday is a struggle to find love and/or keep it. And this ignorance is not just coming in our everyday dealings with each other anymore. It's playing itself out in what we read, what we look at on television, what we listen to on the radio, what we hear at church and what we hear at the local happy hour and group sessions. And we wonder why our society is so upside down.

If my mom were alive she would definitely frown on this concept because she took great pride in the fact that she knew that she was the reason for my dad's success, and not just the beneficiary of it. She knew that she was the reason for my successes in life and not just the **BENEFICIARY!** That is what being a help mate and living up to your true identity as a woman is all about. It is all about being the reason for a man successes and not only the beneficiary. That is why you ridicule each other's desires now, and label them with words like "gold digger" and "needy" because most women have lost their perspective on this interpretation. Your true identity has taken a backseat to motives.

My mom knew that it said just as much about her that my father took on God's interpretation, as it said about him. She took great pride in knowing that she was the catalyst that pushed my stepfather into greatness. She took it as an honor to be the reason for him transforming into a man that knew his true identity through her energy and effort towards that. She even helped me be the best man that I could possibly be. And she did it all with God's interpretation of things. Of course, she would have never been able to teach me or my father how to be the men we turned out to be, on her interpretation of things or society's interpretation of things. But she knew that as long as she brought her true identity to the table that it wouldn't be long before me and my stepfather—as the beneficiaries of her true identity were going to do the same. As a woman, your true identity is the reason for a man's success. And the only way that's going to happen is to start bringing God's interpretation of things to the table so that it resonates with the men in your life.

"Everybody wants to be the solution, but no one wants to be told that they are part of the problem."

Stop being part of your own problem. Live up to your true identity as a woman so that a man can start living up to his. Start taking the initiative to be the reason for a man's success, rather than only the beneficiary of it. Stop allowing society to use scare tactics for you as women not to live up to your calling, so that a man can live up to his. Society has put a heavy burden on you, which was not meant for you—and you bought into the negativity of it all. You have continued to disregard your importance to the general makeup of a man. You are truly vital to his ability to live up to God's interpretation. He will never get the honorable mention that is awarded kings without your input. And you will never get the honorable mention that is awarded to queens without his. One would think this knowledge would put most of you at ease. But I don't want to put you at ease more than put you on guard by saying that...

"If you're not the reason for a man's success, then you will become the excuse for his failures."

That is why I said earlier in this chapter that a man will never leave a woman helping him live up to God's interpretation—because it's not something that every woman is good at, if at all. It's not even something that most women want to do even though they know the truth of it all. That is why a man bringing this interpretation with him is very rare because we do need that woman who says she is ready to live up to her true identity so she can help us live up to ours. It's a lost art, but it can be found again. We as men and women just have to know where to look! And what better place to look than inward and upward!

I have to be honest and say that the reason I am so adamant about this concept is because I was one of those men who by his own admission didn't live up to God's interpretation of things because I felt that society would make it their mission to discredit me even if they couldn't discredit what I am writing. But as I wrote earlier, I can no longer live by a woman's or society's desire to keep me in the past, and would say to you not to allow this blatant disrespect for your calling to go on as well. Be the man or the woman that you always knew you were. It's a wise investment of your belief system to accept the fact that your true identity has never left you, and that you have left your true identity behind. Look yourself in the mirror and know that you have always been more than good enough for God. And last but not least—someone is out there waiting for you to inspire, motivate or encourage them to be what you have always claimed you wanted, and it will find its way into your life and your heart.

CHAPTER 9

Evolution to Ignorance

Since the beginning of time women have been making their case to not only be seen but heard, and it couldn't be more evident than it is today in our society where women are no longer taking a back-seat to men. Tired of being taken for granted by the rules and regulation that only benefited men in the past, women have begun to fight for their right to exist in a man's world. It has been a tiresome crusade to say the least, but for the most part, women have found their identity and are letting man know about it every chance they get.

I can't say that I remember a lot from the 1970's as a youth about the way women were treated because I grew up with a mom who was more like the women of today more than the women I read about when I did my research before writing this chapter. Growing up during that time, I was the beneficiary of a fight that started a long time before I had the right to exist. And with that being said, I take my position in this world now with a greater appreciation than I had in my 20's and early 30's. And so! It is for this reason that I now bring the fight back to you, the reader, to understand how evolution has turned into ignorance. But not before I bring up two of the most prominent women who were the catalyst for that evolution.

Susan B. Anthony and Elizabeth Cady Stanton

These were two of the first women to fight for the equalities and freedoms of not only women, but anyone they felt was being treating unfairly by the laws of this land. But I will just focus on the female aspect of this story for now. When I decided to write this chapter, I told myself that I was going to be sympathetic to the history of the evolution these women brought on by doing some research about how this evolution came about before I decided to give my interpretation of how it has become ignorant. I wanted to be fair in my observation and respectful to these women so my opinions and findings wouldn't come off like I was disregarding history while presenting my case.

Too be honest, I had no idea what was in store for me when I began reading about these two women. But I couldn't wait to find out about their story. And I must say that I was extremely impressed with their dedication to women's rights, as I embark on my dedication towards man's arguments about women's rights. I was extremely impressed with their ability to make their case with men without using words or phrases that would give these men a misinterpretation to go on. But you have to follow me to understand what I mean.

Oftentimes, when I hear today's women speak on their rights to be independent and self-sufficient, they seem to come off as angry and unattractive instead of articulate and beautiful. Their personal style comes across as brash and unapproachable more than classy and gentle. And even though I agree with most women about the things that have made women look inferior to men, I still feel that doing it in a lady like way goes a lot further than doing it like you're a woman who is still in the 1900's. And no, I don't mean bringing on an interpretation to man that you're weak or scared, but instead, bringing an approach to the table that doesn't allow us as men to see your point more than your rage about your point.

"I would define that as bringing an attitude that doesn't render a good result, but expecting a good result."

As I read up on Susan B. Anthony, I came to know that she was an extremely bright woman. But she was also a very brass and outspoken woman and was not afraid to debate with men about the issues women faced because she had the articulation and the where with all to do so. She had the ability and the desire. She had the conviction and the knowledge. She would have definitely been one of the most revered women if she were alive today, bringing her fight to the masses. In a sense, I wish she was alive today because I know that she would not have let the women of today turn her evolution into ignorance. I couldn't imagine how she would feel or how any other woman would feel back then about how women have taken their right to be treated the way they wanted all along and then turn it back into a man's favor.

I mean….. I would think that women have become smarter as time has gone on. I would think that women would have evolved at a more rapid pace than they are now. I would even think that as women you would make sure you said or did nothing that would give men the indication that you have no clue on how to be treated by a man. But I see it too often than I care to admit. I see too often that women have said and done things that have given man the indication that everything these women fought for in the past means nothing to them. That everything that has transpired means nothing to them because most of them don't understand how they have taken evolution and made it ignorant.

Now before I started doing my research for this chapter, I would hear the ramblings and arguments from women about how men treated women back then and to be honest! I thought to myself "It couldn't have been that bad" until I started reading about these women that I would later have a greater respect for. I was very ashamed because I had allowed a woman's evolution to even bring out the ignorance in me because I live in an era where women are not being taken for granted the way they were in the past. It wasn't until I looked beyond my own ignorance, did I start to understand why women are so adamant about being "Independent" or "Self sufficient". It wasn't until I looked beyond my own ignorance did I start to understand how important it has been for women to make their own way in life. I mean! Who am I to say that a woman doesn't have a right to feel this way? I mean! Who am I to say that women don't have a right to want the best out of a man! Who am I to tell them that their issues and opinions about men are not valid because they are!

But as time has gone on, I have gotten very familiar with the way women approach men these days. And I have to wonder if most women know what evolution's point was to them getting everything they desired out of men. I wonder if most women know what Susan B. Anthony's point was when fighting for their rights to have a voice. Susan B. Anthony's point about evolution did not start with an economic mentality or argument towards how women were being treated in the work place. Susan B. Anthony's point about evolution started because of the way husbands treated wives, and father's treated daughters. It started with the things she saw as a woman personally.

This is based on a true story:

When Susan B. Anthony was in her teens, her father owned a sewing company and she frequented there often. One day while working there, she would later find her cause through a personal situation with her father. Her father was looking for someone to fill the managerial position at his company, and Susan felt like she knew just the person who was more qualified than any other person to have that job. So she went to her father and mentioned this woman's name, who was the best seamstress her father had working for him. No one knew more about sewing or had more knowledge about sewing than this woman, who Susan had recommended for the job. But being the way that men were back then about women being in managerial jobs, her dad settled on a man that was less qualified than the woman Susan felt should have gotten the job. It made Susan furious that her own father was using gender to stop this woman who was more qualified than the man he hired, from getting the position. Even though Susan B. Anthony would later go out into the world to make an economic argument about the way women were treated back then, it was her personal issues about her dad's approach that brought on that argument.

Here it is women are making their argument about being "Independent" on an economic point when it is your personal life that you are suffering from. As women, you are making it seem like to men that all you are struggling with is the economic part of your life. That is why we as men have jumped on that "Independent" bandwagon because we think that if a woman's only issue when we meet her is an economic issue then we're good as men. If a woman's only issue is that a man is not stepping up to the plate financially and she has already taken care of that problem, we are in the clear. There are so many things that I see women these days struggling with and it always fascinates me that none of these things are being brought up in their dealings with men to justify why they are "Independent".

Most of those issues never even make its way into a conversation with a man because society has told you that a man doesn't want to hear about your personal issues. But it's not your personal issues we have no interest in. It is the stories about your ex boyfriend and all the other guys that you had these personal issues with that we have no interest in you sharing. As men, we feel like we can help you with the issues that you are struggling with. But we can't help with the issues that you are struggling with about some other man. And the moment a man feels like he can't help you or he is helpless to your situation and issues that is when he will start to question his desire to move forward with you. That is when he will start to see that your evolution may end up turning the situation into ignorance.

I mean.... as women, some of you have to know or should know that it doesn't make me or any man feel like much for going out of our way to please a woman who comes at us with their evolution to ignorance type of mentality to think that we are going to meet your needs or even learn how to meet your needs when you're dissolving right before our eyes. And no, we don't understand what you mean by telling us that you're an independent woman because you're only making that argument based on one argument when there are so many other things that you women are struggling with in your personal life as opposed to your economic one. That's why I don't understand how you can continue to make your arguments based on society's way of seeing things. I don't understand how you think that as women bringing on an economic argument to justify your personal issues is ever going to get your personal needs met.

And it is up to us as men not to allow this to keep happening. As men, we should be telling them that we are no longer going to allow them to make an economic argument to justify their personal issues with us anymore. It is up to us as men not to allow society to help women justify their ignorance by making a point about evolution that has nothing to do with the way you as men are going to go about meeting their needs. Women are making an economic argument that has nothing to do with how a man is going to go about meeting their personal needs. And you wonder why men as a whole are not being responsible for your emotions. But you never made your "Independent" argument about emotions. You wonder why he is not being responsible for your sex life. But you never made your "Independent" argument about sex. You wonder why he isn't being responsible for your children. But you never made your "Independent" argument about your children. So how do you expect for a man to be responsible for all these other elements about you when you're not making your arguments based on any of those things? You have to understand as women that….

"Man is going on the definition of the word "Independent", while women are going on the interpretation of the word "Independent"

You have to understand that if you're not going to make your arguments about all the other elements in your life, then don't expect for a man to try and be responsible for them. Don't expect for a man to just automatically know that these things need taking care of when nothing about your approach towards men has made him feel like these things are even important to you. He never even knew that these things existed. But a man that knows that these things are important to you will always be aware of those things because contrary to what society has told you....

"A man will never deny you of the desires he agreed upon from the START!"

He will never deny you because his intentions were for you to fill him in on how he can be successful with your way of doing things. He will never deny you of anything as long as he is included. One of the things out of the many things that I respected about Susan B. Anthony was her keen sense to understand that she was going to make her arguments for women in all aspects of life, and not just economically. It was never a fight economically for her. It was a fight about the right to be **INCLUDED**! But this "Independent" woman approach that women are on today was not brought on by evolution. It was brought on by the ignorance of some to speak on how evolution was going to bridge the gap between men and women. But as far as I'm concerned it has done no such thing.

Now I'm almost sure that when Susan B. Anthony and Elizabeth Cady Stanton fought for women's rights, there would be a lot that they would be proud of, and well they should be. But I'm sure that there would be a lot that they are not proud of. When I look at our world today I find that it's hard separating the boys from the men. In the same way, it is hard separating the women from the girls. And more confusing is the fact that we sometimes can't accept one without the other. But I have to be fair about the fact that our world has become almost all about evolution that will always bring on a certain kind of ignorance.

"We have used our own reasons and desires to ruin ourselves."

We have used our own motives and purposes to fuel the ignorance of others. We have used our tongues and demeanors to offend the conscious mind by helping people make excuses for their actions in the unconscious mind. Not only are we not taking responsibility for the ignorance that has been brought on by evolution, we are not even holding people accountable for the way they fuel that ignorance in others. My greatest satisfaction and reward comes through my ability to make things easier for a woman. It has and will always be the thing that I am graded on in this life and in heaven. Most women do not realize that you are taking away man's greatest satisfaction and reward with your independence.

You don't realize that evolution has not made things easier for you. If anything it has made things much harder for you. And I understand the reason behind wanting to be able to pay your own way when you go on a date so that a man doesn't try to subject or obligate you to something you're not ready for. I understand that you don't want to have to go through the ringer to get your hair and nails done by your man. I understand all of that! But what I don't understand is how most women come at men from the start with this evolution to ignorance mentality that you are self-sufficient and don't need him to do anything. But the minute he has taken your words in its truest form and doesn't do those things, you're mad. Why do you feel that you can come at a man with this evolution to ignorance type approach and still get your needs met? Why do you feel that you can continue to come at us with this self-sufficient mentality and have us not acknowledge it as such? Why do you feel that you can get mad at men for taking your words literal when nothing about your approach said anything that would give us the indication that's not what you really meant?

Here is a news flash for women: the reason why Susan B. Anthony and the women like her back then were never taken for granted by men is because they said what they meant and meant what they said. They didn't leave it up to the men to interpret for them because they knew it would never benefit them or any other woman for that matter. That was the most disheartening thing to Susan B. Anthony that women were allowing men to do this in the first place. In the words of Susan B. Anthony, she writes:

"It is the disheartening part of my life that so few women will work for the emancipation of their own half of the race…. very few are capable of seeing that the cause of nine tenths of all the misfortunes which come to women, and to men, lies in the subjective of women."

When I read this quote by Susan B. Anthony, I was not only taken back by her authentic willingness to challenge women back then to see that they were the root cause of their own sufferings when it came to being respected by men, but those words still apply to today's women as well. Whether it's the "independent woman" approach, daytime television or all the children who are being raised in single parent homes these days, very few women will ever see that the cause of nine tenths of all the misfortunes which come to women, and to men, lies in the subjective of women. Now I know you're asking yourself, what does that mean, Tonee? Well…. just for your sake and mine, I went online and looked up the definition of the word subjective, which I believe best matches against what Susan B. Anthony meant by her quote.

"SUBJECTIVE:" Existing in the mind, belonging to the thinking subject, rather than the object of thought.

What Susan B. Anthony was saying is that it was disheartening to her to see a woman allowing the men in their lives to think for them and then not object to the fact that his way of thinking was not going to meet their everyday needs. And I would agree with her. I would agree that no woman should ever allow a man or mate to think for her or try to interpret how she gets her needs met. But what I don't agree with is how women have used evolution to make excuses that men are not living up to their billing. But you have to follow me to understand where I am going with this point. Now with regard to evolution and the ignorance it has caused since the Susan B. Anthony's and Elizabeth Cady Stanton's have made their way through history, one of the things that have always puzzled me about our society is how we take no stock in what women say in certain instances but we take stock in others. Not only did we not take a lot of stock in what women said back then, we still don't take much stock in what women say today. But you have to follow me to understand how evolution has turned to ignorance.

When Susan B. Anthony was trying to get man to take stock in what she was saying about women's rights back then, men were not trying to listen. She accepted full responsibility for what she said back in those days, even if society didn't want to. Now that evolution has come along and provided women with the "voice" that Susan B. Anthony fought for—it seems that not only have women become ignorant with that voice, but they have not been held responsible for that ignorance it has caused in men. I know! It comes as a shocker to you as women that I said this. But you won't be shocked in a minute when I present you with the reason. Now that evolution has made its way into the consciousness, men definitely take stock in what women say these days because we know that if we didn't take stock in what women said we would get labeled for not doing so.

The catch 22 in it is this: too often I hear women telling men what they believe is going to give them the best chance to succeed with making their point of being "Independent". And more often than not, it is the point that you really don't need us in order for you to make your way in this life. But what you don't understand as women is not only has man taken stock in what you just said, he is going to make sure that you are the one who is held responsible for the words that are coming out of your mouth, even if society is not. Man is going to make sure that you are responsible for the "interpretation" while he goes on the "definition" of your words. We as men have allowed women to turn evolution into ignorance. We have allowed women to not only object to our way of thinking and doing things our way, but most of you are not even taking responsibility for the fact that they have sabotaged men being included. As women you don't understand that it is not man that is stopping you from winning your case against us. It is the approach that I spoke of in the previous paragraph that is stopping you women from winning your case against us. It's like….

"A lawyer who objects to an idea brought on by another attorney against his client, but then uses his grounds to make the other attorney's case for him"

You women out there in society have gone from evolution to ignorance. You don't realize that you are objecting to man's way of treating you, but then using your grounds to stop a man from meeting your needs. You should be objective on the grounds that man is not meeting your needs. Not objecting on the grounds that you're an independent woman. I know that your intention was for this whole thing to benefit you. And it may well be benefiting you in your professional life. That doesn't mean that it will benefit you in your personal life. The reason why man will never take a chance on a woman that has taken him from evolution to ignorance is because he feels that you will never appreciate him taking on his responsibility for that part of your life that is giving him his greatest satisfaction and reward. Man is saying that…

"You can have your cake and eat it too!"

But as history has shown, most women look at this as a set up instead of a benefit. You look at it as a rail-roading instead of a perk. You look at it as a man trying to control you instead of a man trying to give you as many options as you could possibly want in order to make your case with society and the people around you. Society has once again sold you on this concept that people only want to help you when you can help yourself. But what society forgot to tell you is that they are only helping you because they see a benefit. Therefore, if there was no benefit to helping you help yourself, society wouldn't even help you. Or better yet, if your ability to help yourself didn't take away society's benefiting anyway, they still wouldn't help you. But a man doesn't see it that way. He knows where his benefit comes from. And that's seeing you happy as you meet his being desired by you as well. We as men don't want to be left out of our benefits or blessings either. So we will never be with a woman who is not only using evolution to bring on ignorance towards that, but not taking responsibility for doing so. Please tell me how you can be mad at a man for not meeting the needs you claim you can meet yourself? And why do you think that means that he should be doing it because you can do it for yourself? Like I said in my earlier chapters…

"You do it yourselfers are going to be by yourselfers"

Men are telling you that you can have your cake and eat it too—as long as you are coming at us with the understanding that we take stock in what comes out of your mouth. In addition, you need to be responsible for what you say to us. Society will always give you an excuse and have you thinking that the way that you're coming at men is correct, so they can continue to profit from your ignorance. It's time to grow up ladies! It's time for you to start getting mad at those women who are giving man the indication that you're all the same and start challenging them to see that evolution has not made you ignorant or naïve.   Women need to understand that men take a lot of stock in what you say to them from the start. Your mouth piece is your greatest commodity. I suggest you start using it as such and start acting like a woman that understands that

"Being a woman is not doing a man's job. Being a woman is getting a man to do it!"

And if you as a woman cannot get a man to be responsible for you, then I feel that you are telling me and the rest of the world that your game is weak. And you need to step your game up. GOD gave you an undeniable ability to get you needs met by men. So why don't you start using it. Quit allowing society to tell you that you don't have the ability to get a man to do any and everything you need him to do. Quit letting society make it seem like your desires are brought on by weakness and not strengths. They have already taken away your sex appeal and beauty and made it a negative aspect of being you. They have already taken away your desire to have a man making things easier for you while replacing it with a work ethic and responsibility that has you doing things harder than you ever have before.

It's sad to see that women have given up on men so easily and so quickly. And if you're going to keep bringing evolution to the table to justify your ignorance with men then do me a favor and apologize to those women who came before you who have given you the right to have a "voice." You owe it to them to start acting like the women they felt they were fighting for so that we as men can start living up to the billing.

The greatest gift and the greatest tragedy that God ever gave man was a WOMAN!

So which one are you going to be?

CPSIA information can be obtained at www.ICGtesting.com
Printed in the USA
BVOW010303101212

307662BV00006B/13/P